THE GIRL
WHO GAVE
BIRTH
TO RABBITS

Works by Clifford A. Pickover

The Alien IQ Test

Black Holes: A Traveler's Guide

Chaos and Fractals

Chaos in Wonderland

Computers, Pattern, Chaos, and Beauty

Computers and the Imagination

Cryptorunes

Future Health: Computers and Medicine in the 21st Century

Fractal Horizons: The Future Use of Fractals

Frontiers of Scientific Visualization (with Stu Tewksbury)

Keys to Infinity

The Loom of God

Mazes for the Mind: Computers and the Unexpected

The Pattern Book: Fractals, Art, and Nature

The Science of Aliens

Spider Legs (with Piers Anthony)

Spiral Symmetry (with Istvan Hargittai)

Strange Brains and Genius

Surfing Through Hyperspace

Time: A Traveler's Guide

Visions of the Future

Visualizing Biological Information

Wonders of Numbers

CLIFFORD A. PICKOVER, PH.D.

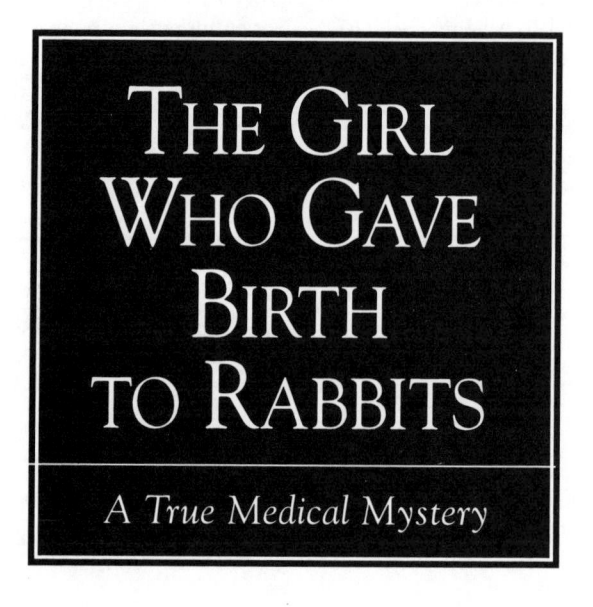

THE GIRL WHO GAVE BIRTH TO RABBITS

A True Medical Mystery

Prometheus Books

59 John Glenn Drive
Amherst, New York 14228-2197

Published 2000 by Prometheus Books

Inquiries should be addressed to
Prometheus Books, 59 John Glenn Drive, Amherst, New York 14228–2197.
VOICE: 716–691–0133, ext. 207.
FAX: 716–564–2711.
WWW.PROMETHEUSBOOKS.COM

04 03 02 01 00   5 4 3 2 1

Library of Congress Cataloging-in-Publication Data

Pickover, Clifford A.
    The girl who gave birth to rabbits : a true medical mystery / by Clifford A. Pickover.
        p.   cm.
    Includes bibliographical references and index.
    ISBN 1–57392–794–5 (alk. paper)
    1. Toft, Mary 1701–1763—Health. 2. Abnormalities, Human. 3. Medical misconceptions. I. Title.
RG627 .P53 1999
618.2—dc21
[B]   99–056193
                                                                                                          CIP

Printed in the United States of America on acid-free paper

For the Lagomorpha

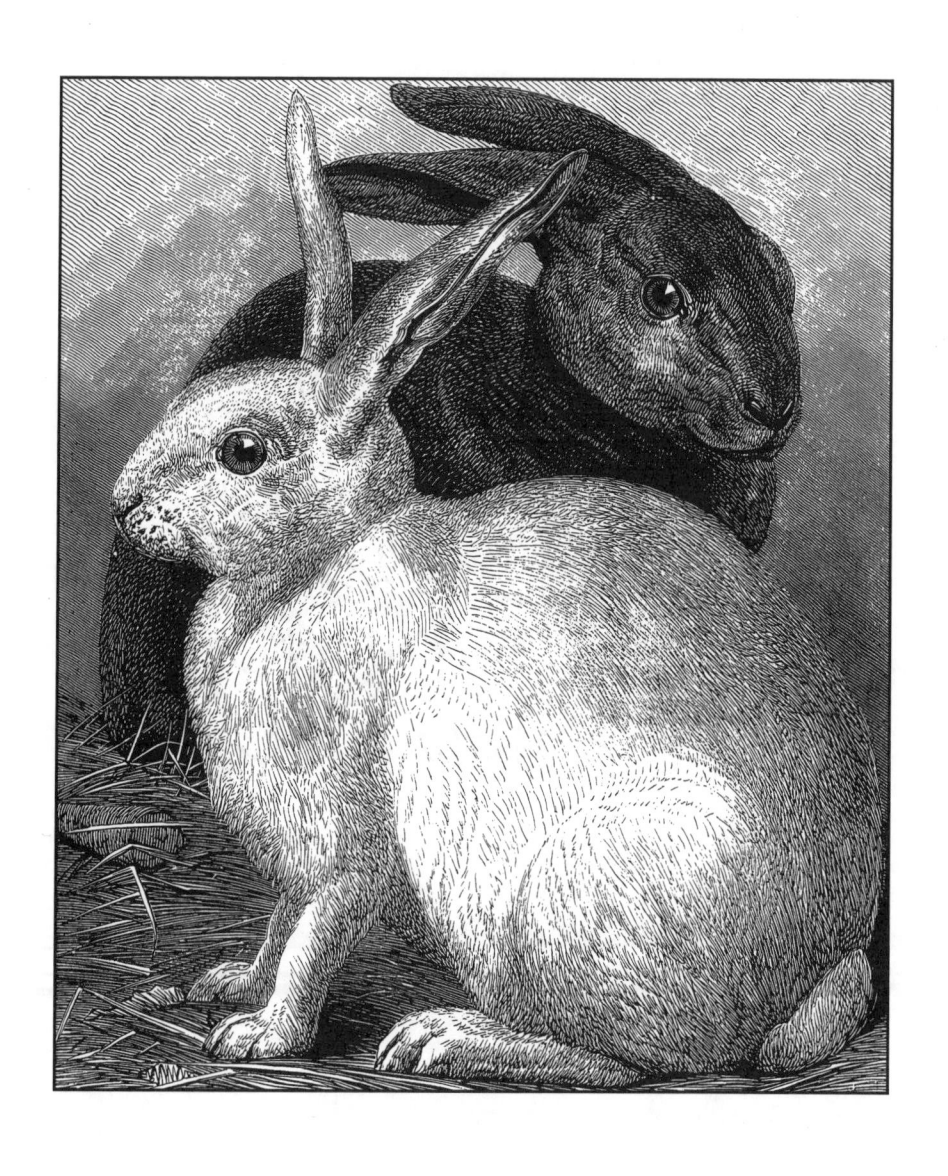

Everything that deceives
may be said to enchant.

—Plato

Plato is dear to me,
but dearer still is truth.

—Aristotle

What matters in the world
is not so much what is true
as what is entertaining,
at least so long as
the truth itself
is unknowable.

—Pierre Larousse

Whosoever lieth with a beast
shall surely be put to death

—Exodus 12:19

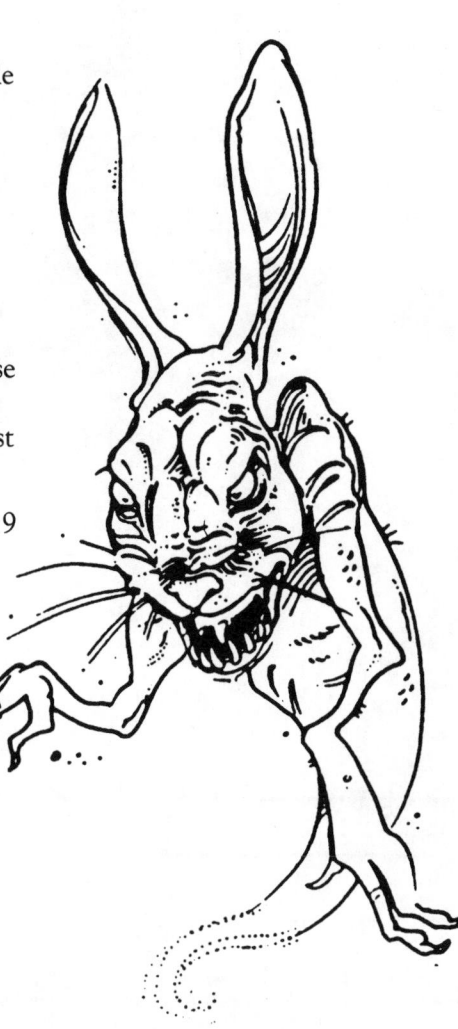

CONTENTS

LIST OF ILLUSTRATIONS

ACKNOWLEDGMENTS

Recently, an exhibition of biological oddities was held in Russia. . . . freakish things afloat in jars. The celebrated anatomist's work was limited to children, infants taken before the age of baptism—the tender veins infused with wax, flesh still fresh with life's last breath. I felt I was a child of the jars. . . . And I never assumed that any tempest could stir me—placid, passive, and eloquent—under glass in my preservative sea.
> —Greg Bills, *Fearful Symmetry*

One of the reasons why religions seems irrelevant today is that many of us no longer have the sense that we are surrounded by the unseen.
> —Karen Armstrong, *A History of God*

I OWE A SPECIAL DEBT OF GRATITUDE TO DENNIS TODD AND Jan Bondeson, both experts on the Mary Toft mystery, for their wonderful past books from which I have drawn many facts about women giving birth to animals and other monstrous things. I heartily recommend their books *Imagining Monsters* and *A Cabinet of Medical Curiosities* for further information on the wonderful Mary Toft. I thank David Glass and Lorraine Miro for useful comments and encouragement.

The illustrations on the deciation page and this page are from Jim Harter, *Animals: A Pictorial Archive of Nineteenth-Century Sources* (New York: Dover, 1979), p. 88, fig. 381. The illustration on the page facing the contents is by April Pedersen for Clifford Pickover.

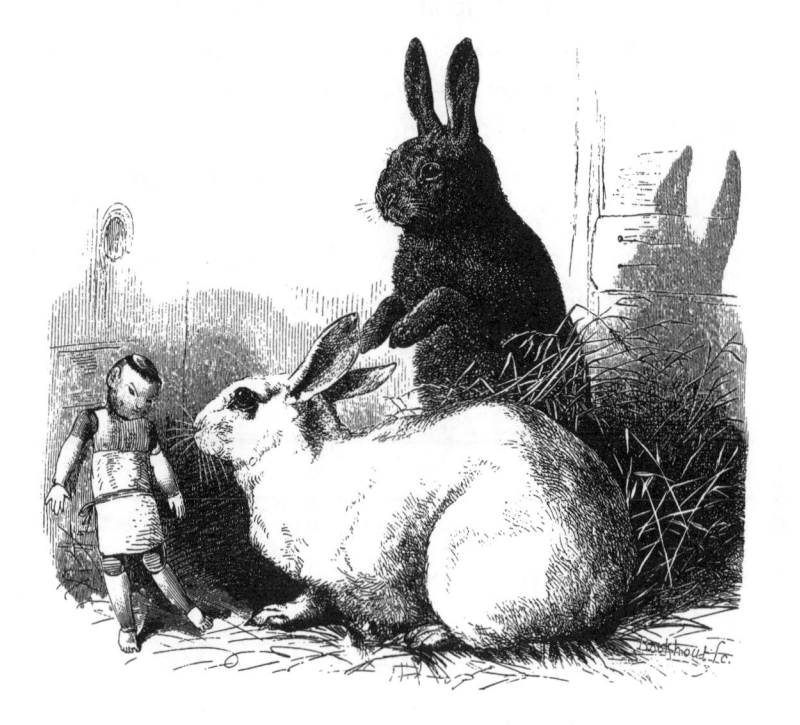

INTRODUCTION

As the island of knowledge grows, the surface that makes contact with mystery expands. When major theories are overturned, what we thought was certain knowledge gives way, and knowledge touches upon mystery differently. This newly uncovered mystery may be humbling and unsettling, but it is the cost of truth. Creative scientists, philosophers, and poets thrive at this shoreline.

—W. Mark Richardson,
"A Skeptic's Sense of Wonder"

Scientists are the easiest to fool. They think in straight, predictable, directable, and therefore misdirectable, lines. The only world they know is the one where everything has a logical explanation and things are what they appear to be. Children and conjurers—they terrify me. Scientists are no problem; against them I feel quite confident.

—James P. Hogan,
Zambendorf: Code of the Lifemaker

And the rabbit, because he cheweth the cud, but divideth not the hoof; he is unclean unto you.

—Leviticus, 11:6

MARY TOFT WAS A YOUNG WOMAN WITH A PECULIAR passion—and an ordinary life that was changed forever when she gave birth to something nonhuman. From that moment onward, she was propelled into a world she had never dreamed existed—a dark, alien, medical subculture flourishing in the courts of the king. She careened out of control, a pawn in the hands of the powerful, yet she forced her contemporaries to question their most basic beliefs.

This book is about history's most fascinating medical mystery—a dark, bloody, true-life *Alice in Wonderland*. Some of Mary's doctors believed her births to be hoaxes while others were convinced the births were real. Decades after the births, priests still debated what had actually transpired, and even today we don't have all the answers.

Why should we care today about a poor eighteenth-century girl who gave birth to rabbits and other monstrous misfits? What relevance could she have to our modern, technological, enlightened world? The answer is that Mary's story contains timeless themes: justice and morality, crime and punishment, and science and superstition separated by the flimsiest of curtains. Her true story also involves sex, money, ambition, scapegoats, jealousy, and scandal involving the leaders of nations. Indeed, Mary's story touches on humankinds' greeds and basic fears. Famous reputations were at stake as the contemporary media went wild in an orgy of lurid reporting—at first with amazing stories of Mary's miraculous births, but later with highly charged personal attacks on all involved. In this theater of the absurd, there are no clear saints and sinners, or winners and losers. Many of Mary's handlers could not tell the difference between imposture and truth, or between themselves and the destructive roles they chose to play.

Another reason we should pay close attention to this tale is that it is a metaphor for today's fringe science, from psychic surgery performed without knives to goat-sucking chupacabras,* to people who claim to bend spoons with their minds. *The X-Files* and *The Exorcist* have nothing on the Mary Toft story. Every day in our modern civilization we are still confronted with claims of wonders.

Hoaxes perpetuated in the name of science come in various flavors. On the one hand, there is the April fools' joke or urban legend in which someone tells a funny tale about alli-

---

*In 1995, reports of a bloodthirsty animal known as El Chupacabras ("the goat-sucker") spread from Puerto Rico to Mexico and the southern United States. The large-eyed, reptilian creature reportedly attacked domesticated animals, draining them of their blood. Subsequent research showed that the dead animals were not drained of blood, and stakeouts usually revealed the presence of wild dogs. The story of the supernatural (or extraterrestrial) chupacabras spread largely through mass hysteria and over-enthusiastic media reports.

gators living in sewers or temporary tattoos laced with LSD, or intimate encounters with gerbils.[1] On the other hand, a more serious hoax can destroy an entire line of scholarship or provide an ineffective medical "cure" until the deceit inevitably comes to light. We can learn many lessons from Mary Toft.

Get set for a demented vacation in a London transformed into a world of mystery and imagination. Along the way you'll learn a little eighteenth-century British history. You probably already know that the 1700s were the age of revolution which saw the birth of the United States. But you are less likely to know about some of the odder goings-on described in this book: the legends of *sooterkins*, molelike animals women were said to give birth to if they stayed too close to hot stoves; artists like French Rococo painter Jean-Honoré Fragonard, who constructed sculptures from human cadavers; collectors like Russia's Peter the Great, who hoarded a bizarre penis collection along with the head of his wife's lover; and other tales of medical mischief and mayhem routinely found in the eighteenth century.

I became fascinated by scientific mysteries involving animals when I first heard about the Watters case from Austell, Georgia. In 1953, young Edward Watters bet a friend ten dollars that he'd get his photo in the local newspaper within two weeks. To win the bet, Watters bought a capuchin monkey for fifty dollars, anesthetized it, and killed it by striking the head.

In case you are not familiar with capuchin monkeys, they are among the most intelligent monkeys in the New World, and are named for their caps of hair resembling the cowls of capuchin monks. These round-headed monkeys are stockily built and stand one to two feet tall, with short, fully haired tails. But none of these distinctive hair patterns mattered much to Watters, who shaved off the monkey's fur in an attempt to make the creature unrecognizable—even alien. With help from a few friends, Watters placed the completely shaved monkey in his truck and drove to a desolate region of Highway 78 outside Austell. Next he slammed on his brakes to make skid marks on the road and then placed the monkey in front of his truck to simulate an accident. Within an hour, a police car arrived at the "accident" scene and found the monkey's body. Watters walked aimlessly around the truck so that he would appear to be in shock. As he walked, he chattered about "Martians."

This was all it took to get the world talking. The police informed local authorities who summoned the FBI, U.S. Air Force, and the Georgia Bureau of Investigation. They all converged on Highway 78 to study the area.

There was TV coverage, and Ed Waters got his name in the papers. He told a story of a "glowing thing, settling down and covering half the highway."[2] Fleshy, monkeylike beings had come ambling out of the craft, and he had run over one of them. It was not his fault. He tried to brake in time.

An autopsy of the creature revealed that the Martian was a capuchin monkey, but Watters had finally won the ten-dollar bet with his friend—although it cost him fifty dollars to purchase the monkey!

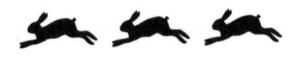

Another animal mystery stimulated my imagination in the mid-1970s. The scene: Puerto Rico's *Laguna Aquas Prietas*—loosely translated as the black lagoon. Alfred Garcia Garameni was swimming when he was suddenly attacked by a bizarre looking creature. The fierce beast was so strong that Garamendi wrestled it, knifed it, and finally shot it several times with his spear gun. The creature was a *garadiavolo*, or "devil fish" (figure 1). Garamendi claimed he had seen a similar four-foot-long creature hopping along the beach several years earlier, but the CIA had taken this first specimen.

Garamendi's preserved his second specimen in a tank. "The creatures are not of this earth," he theorized before the enthralled public and press. "They are from another dimension. They were put here for a purpose. Perhaps for the same reason we might send monkeys and other animals to an alien planet to see how they survive in a strange environment."[3]

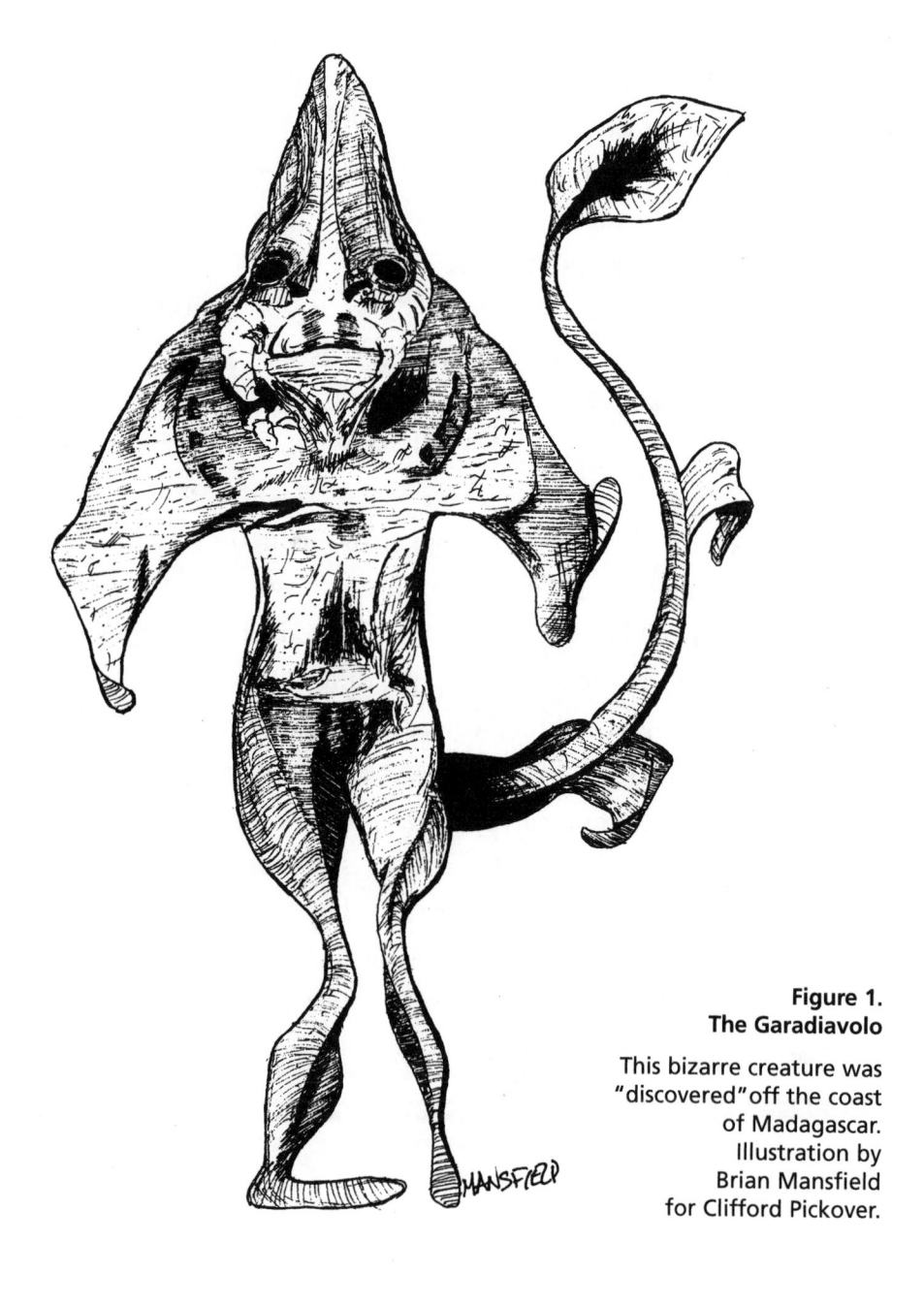

**Figure 1.
The Garadiavolo**

This bizarre creature was "discovered" off the coast of Madagascar. Illustration by Brian Mansfield for Clifford Pickover.

It turned out that Garandendi had actually displayed a guitar fish, a slim-waisted relative of the stringray. In order to make the creature more interesting to look at, he had cut the tail from the fish and moved it. The guitar fish appears to be marked with a devilish human face on its underside. The prominent eyes above the fish's mouths are in fact "nostrils" through which water is exhaled. The creature can be further modified so that it seems to have legs as well as a face.

Through the centuries, the hoaxer has gained a special place in our psyche. Some of these daring mischief-makers have become virtual heroes, even when the hoaxer has perpetrated his fraud for money, revenge, fame, or fun. There was the man who tried to sell the Eiffel Tower for scrap, or the famous Piltdown forgery in which an ape jaw was fitted to a human skull to create a new caveman species. There was also the Cottingley Fairies in which two little girls created fake fairies by using trick photography, or the bogus mammals called "snouters" that used their snouts for walking (figure 2). Then there was the eleven-foot-long Cardiff giant displayed by P. T. Barnam in his legendary circuses (the "giant" was actually a plaster model).

In the last few years, people have become increasingly interested in the paranormal. Television has certainly capital-

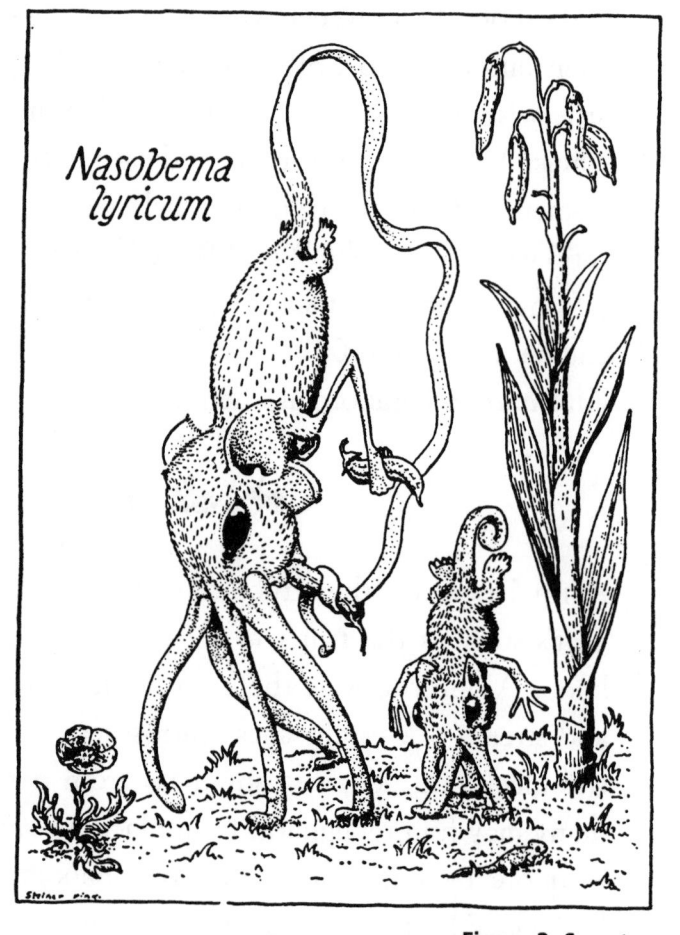

Figure 2. Snouters

These small mammals, known as snouters, evolved remarkable noses for carrying out numerous activities, from walking to grasping and trapping prey. Pictured here are *Nasobema lyricum*, whose snouts are used for walking. When these fanciful animals appeared in an April Fool's Day issue of *Natural History*, some readers believed the creatures to be genuine. From *The Snouters* by Harald Stümpke, translated by Leigh Chadwick (Chicago: University of Chicago Press, 1967), p. 56, plate 10. Translation © 1967 by Doubleday, a division of Bantam Doubleday Dell Publishing Group, Inc. Used by permission of Doubleday, a division of Random House, Inc.

ized on our desire to believe in the strange—everything from alien autopsies, to ESP, to psychic predictions. Even a few otherwise responsible scientists are taken in by some of these scams. With recent surveys indicating that 70 percent of women and 48 percent of men believe in the paranormal,[4] it is no wonder why the World Wide Web also proliferates with information on paranormal phenomena. The Yahoo search engine lists over 1000 such sites under the heading "Science: Alternative: Paranormal Phenomena."[5]

A final note on the structure of this book. Think of Mary Toft's story as the trunk of a tree that runs throughout the book. Along the way, there are various digressive branches and stream-of-consciousness curiosities. This book is not for the meek and does not shy away from describing practices many may find repugnant, from placenta-eating to bestiality. A quote by John Steinbeck, in collaboration with marine biologist Edward Ricketts, sets the tone for the organization of this book:

> The design of a book is the pattern of reality controlled and shaped by the mind of the writer. This is completely understood about poetry or fiction, but is too seldom realized about a book of facts.[6]

If you want an eye-popping mystery, you can quickly read this book, but you will be forever changed as I was when studying the facts of Mary's case. Get set for a roller coaster ride through the wild side of science and human nature. Prepare for a medical merry-go-round. As Winston Churchill said about Russia in 1939, "It is a riddle wrapped in a mystery inside an enigma."

As you read, imagine how Mary's story would play out in modern days, or in centuries before Mary Toft, or even in biblical times. As you read, chant the words that the Lord spoke to Moses in Leviticus. Chant them over and over each time you need constancy, hope, and a firm footing in Mary Toft's shifting universe:

> You shall not let your animals breed with a
>   different kind;
> you shall not sow your field with two kinds
>   of seed;
> nor shall you put on a garment made of two
>   different materials.[7]

NOTES

1. For an interesting website on modern urban legends, see www.urbanlegends.com. Also see the Usenet discussion group alt.folklore.urban.

2. Nick Yapp, *Greatest Hoaxes of the World* (London: Robson Books, 1992)

3. The Editors of Time-Life, *Hoaxes and Deceptions* (New York: Time-Life), pp. 35–36.

4. Benjamin Radford, "Paranormal Belief Survey," *Skeptical Inquirer* 22, no. 2 (March/April 1998): 8.

5. To give you an idea of the range of material on the World Wide Web, we can sort the Yahoo paranormal topics by the number of web pages in each category. (Of course, these numbers change almost daily and only represent a tiny sampling of the entire corpus of websites devoted to the paranormal but not indexed at Yahoo.) Some numbers are approximate because these major headings include subheadings and sub-subheadings, and I did not carefully go through the entire hierarchy to obtain exact counts of all web pages under all subheadings. Naturally some categories overlap.

Companies (523)

Extraterrestrial Life (423)

Astrology (156)

Witchcraft (114)

Magic (87)

Divination (82)

Mysticism (71)

Skeptics (46)

Ghosts (43)

Cryptozoology (33)

Parapsychology (23)

Horror (22)

Magazines (19)

Organizations (18)

Voodoo (18)

Crop Circles (16)

End of Millennium (16)

Near-Death Experiences (16)

Occult (14)

Parody (14)

Astral Projection (12)

Loch Ness (11)

Kirlian Photography (10)

Ancient Civilizations (9)

Reincarnation (8)
Alchemy (7)
Dowsing (7)
Regional Guides (7)
Spiritism (7)
Remote Viewing (7)
Bell, Art (7)
Luck (6)
Biorhythm (6)

Healings (5)
Hollow Earth (5)
Spontaneous Human Combustion (5)
Chat (4)
Personal Experience (4)
Usenet (4)
Bermuda Triangle (2)

Note that the "Extraterrestrial Life" category is dominated not by scientific speculation but by topics such as Roswell, aliens, and close encounters. The "Companies" category deals with such topics as astrology, tarot, numerology, and other psychic phenomena. It would be fascinating to see how these numbers and categories change through time.

We can focus on a particular category, "Cryptozoology," indexed by the Yahoo search engine. (The number of sites in this category had roughly doubled in the few months since I catalogued the general paranomal category.) The major Cryptozoology categories include Bigfoot (22 sites), Loch Ness Monster (12) and Chupacabra (10), followed by a host of other unusual topics such as Goatmen, Bat Boy, the Altamaha-Ha of Georgia, Nguio Rung (Vietnamese forest people), the elusive Drop Bears from Australia, Storsjon Lake monsters in Sweden, Beasts of Bodmin Moor (large animals said to be in Britain), and the Zuiyo-maru Carcass from New Zealand (supposed by some to be a plesiosaur). In case you are not familiar with some of the lesser-known creatures, Bat Boy is a half-human, half-bat said to have been found in a West Virginia underworld. The Altamaha-Ha is a large, dark water-creature named after the river it frequents, the Altamaha. The local newspaper, *The Darien News*, has recorded a number of sightings. Darien, Georgia is a small fishing town in McIntosh county, which is veined with waterways and protected from the sea by barrier islands.

Some of the websites are humorous and include lurid photos. Others are clearly unskeptical about the creatures they describe. A few sites mention the scientific side of cryptozoology, which is the study of newly discovered and rediscovered organisms, and hypothetical creatures thought to exist based on the biological clues they leave behind. While the field is famous for controversial monsters like the Loch Ness, Sasquatch, and Mokele-Mbembe (the supposedly living dinosaur), cryptozoology includes the scientific study of inconspicuous insects and invertebrates.

One scientific example of a crytpozoological find is the okapi, a short-necked giraffe mentioned in the 1890 book *In Darkest Africa*, but not officially recognized by the scientific community until 1901. The mountain gorilla was reported by an explorer in 1860 but wasn't officially recognized until 1902. Other examples abound.

Cryptozoology also deals with animals that are believed to be extinct, but nevertheless could still roam the Earth. Consider the coelacanth, thought to be an extinct fish only found in the fossil record, but in 1938 a live specimen was caught off the coast of southern Africa.

In the early 90s, the Vu Quang Nature Reserve in Vietnam was a hotbed of cryptozoological finds. In 1992, a new fish, bird, turtle, and large mammal were found. The large mammal is called the Vu Quang ox, known locally as Sao La. Previously, scientists had only found a few horns, skulls, and skin samples, although there were anecdotal reports from hunters about living Vu Quang ox. In June of 1994, Vietnamese scientists finally captured a five-month-old calf.

The term "cryptozoology" was coined by Dr. Bernard Heuvelmans in his personal correspondence to colleagues in the 1950s, after the 1955 French publication of his book *On the Track of Unknown Animals*.

6. John Steinbeck and Edward Flanders Ricketts, *The Log from the Sea of Cortez* (New York: Penguin, 1995).

7. Leviticus 19:1–18.

CAST OF CHARACTERS

Science is not about control. It is about cultivating a perpetual condition of wonder in the face of something that forever grows one step richer and subtler than our latest theory about it. It is about reverence, not mastery.
—Richard Powers, *The Gold Bug Variations*

IN ORDER OF APPEARANCE

Mary Toft	the girl who gave birth to rabbits
Joshua Toft	Mary's husband, an unsuccessful cloth-worker
Mary Gill	the Tofts' neighbor
Ann Toft	Mary's mother-in-law; a midwife.
John Howard	"midwife" of the town of Guildford
King George I	King of Great Britain

Nathanael St. André	surgeon from London
Samuel Molyneux	Secretary to Prince of Wales, Royal Society Fellow
Mrs. Mason	owned the Guildford house where Mary stayed
Mary Costen	attended Mary while in Guildford
Margaret Toft	Mary's sister-in-law
Cyriacus Ahlers	German surgeon on staff to King George
Lord John Hervey	an English politician
Sir Richard Manningham	one of the greatest obstetricians of Mary's time
Sooterkins	molelike animals believed to be born from Dutch women who stayed too close to hot stoves.
Dr. John Maubray	a London obstetrician who believed in sooterkins (see above).
James Douglas	famous surgeon specializing in female organs
Dr. Limborsch	German obstetrician present at the bathhouse
Thomas Brathwait	a famous surgeon present at the bathhouse
Thomas Howard	porter at the bathhouse

Sir Thomas Clarges   justice of the peace, investigator of Mary

Lord Thomas Onslow   justice of the peace, investigator of Mary

LOCATIONS

Act I. Godalming, England
Act II. Guildford, England
Act III. Leicester Fields and London, England

TIMELINE (AUGUST–DECEMBER 1726)

August	September	October	November	December
Mary's Miscarriage	First Monstrous Catlike Birth	Rabbit Births	St. André in Guildford	Mary in Bathhouse; Mary in prison

Chapter One

In the Beginning

All scientific knowledge that we have of this world, or will ever have, is as an island in the sea of mystery. We live in our partial knowledge as the Dutch live on polders claimed from the sea. We dike and fill. We dredge up soil from the bed of mystery and build ourselves room to grow. . . . Scratch the surface of knowledge and mystery bubbles up like a spring. And occasionally, at certain disquieting moments in history (Aristarchus, Galileo, Planck, Einstein), a tempest of mystery comes rolling in from the sea and overwhelm our efforts.

—Chet Raymo,
Honey from Stone: A Naturalist's Search for God

*The real power of Mary Toft—whether it lay in her ability
to convert a human fetus into an animal, to provoke
sexual desire, or to make a man a fool—was to draw man
lower than he was, to make him a beast in some way, to
transform him downward to the body.*
　　　　　　　　—Dennis Todd, *Imagining Monsters*

*When the stars threw down their spears
And water'd heaven with their tears,
Did he smile his work to see?
Did he who made the Lamb make thee?*
　　　　　　　　—William Blake, "The Tyger"

MARY TOFT GAVE BIRTH TO HER FIRST RABBIT IN October of 1726. Soon a nation would be enthralled, prominent medical men would be baffled, and even King George I of Great Britain would demand an official investigation. Although the king would die the following year, he would live to understand the full extent of this medical enigma.

I can hear you wondering out loud. How did she do it? Doesn't it violate the laws of science? Was it a hoax? Could it be her baby was a human child with a birth defect giving it rabbitlike features?

Let's set the scene. Imagine yourself transported to the rustic village of Godalming in the county of Surrey, England

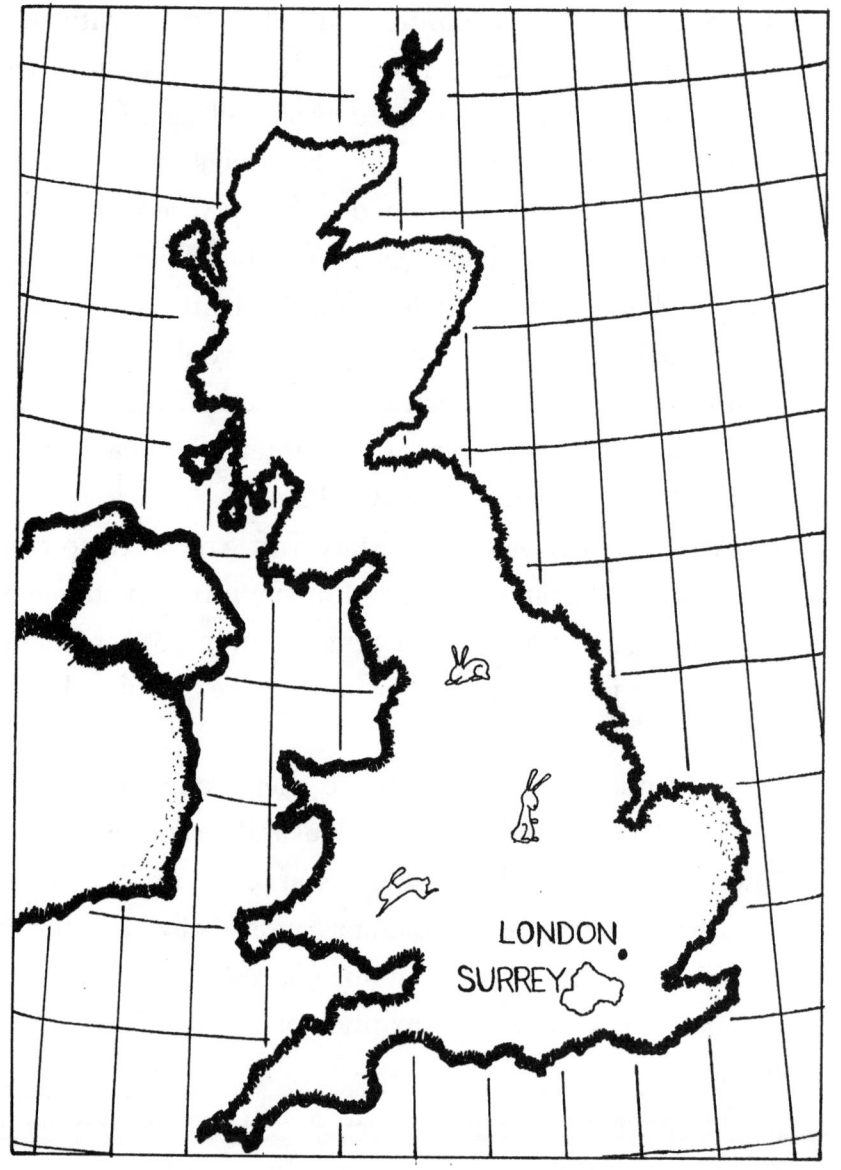

Figure 3. Surrey, England

Illustration by Brian Mansfield for Clifford Pickover.

(figure 3). Today, Godalming is full of churches with twisted spires, timbered buildings from the 1800s, and narrow streets, most of which can be negotiated by a small car. Situated south of London in the valleys of the rivers Wey and Ock, Godalming was first mentioned in King Alfred's[1] will in 880 C.E. By 1086, the village was relatively affluent. The town prospered during the Middle Ages, and by the sixteenth century Godalming became a center of the wool and cloth trade. Business flourished through the Elizabethan times up to the 1700s, when foreign competition intensified and made life more difficult for the citizens Godalming.

About twenty years *after* Mary Toft gave birth to rabbits, the main road from London to Portsmouth opened—making Godalming a convenient stopping place. In 1881, Godalming became the first town in the world to have a public electricity supply.

Continue to imagine you are there today. Look around you. Smell the fresh honeysuckle and lavender. From the town, across the River Wey, you can see bright green meadows known as the Lammaslands. Following the river north you come to the tranquil Catteshall Lock and Farncombet House where all manner of boats are available for hire.

The year is 1726. Imagine twenty-five-year-old Mary Toft, the heroine of our strange story. She's been married to her husband, Joshua, for six years. Of their three children, two are still alive. Their names are Mary and James. Anne, who was born in March 1723, died four months later from smallpox. James is two and was born in July 1724. His sister Mary's exact date of birth is unknown. The following family tree should help clarify this.

THE TOFT FAMILY TREE

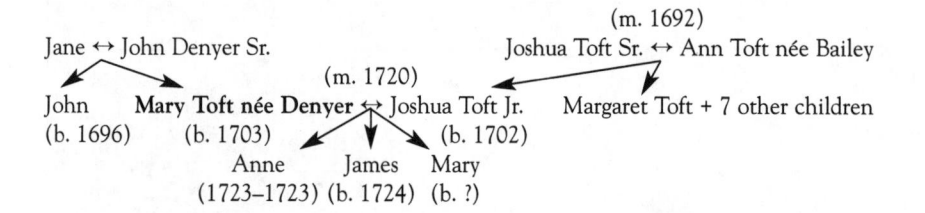

The Toft ancestors had lived in bucolic Godalming since the early 1600s, and most of the generations had made a good living in the woolen trade. However, by the 1720s the Tofts were living in harder times. Mary's husband, Joshua, was a poorly paid laborer who was hired to cut and finish cloth. As an unsuccessful journeyman clothier (cloth-worker), Joshua didn't have the money for his family to live in high style, eat good food, or have the fancy clothes of earlier Tofts.

The literature describes Mary as being short, stout, with coarse features, and of a "stupid and sullen temper."[2] However, you should take such reports with a grain of salt because they may be colored by eighteenth-century attitudes toward unsophisticated women (figure 4). Nathanael St. André, a surgeon

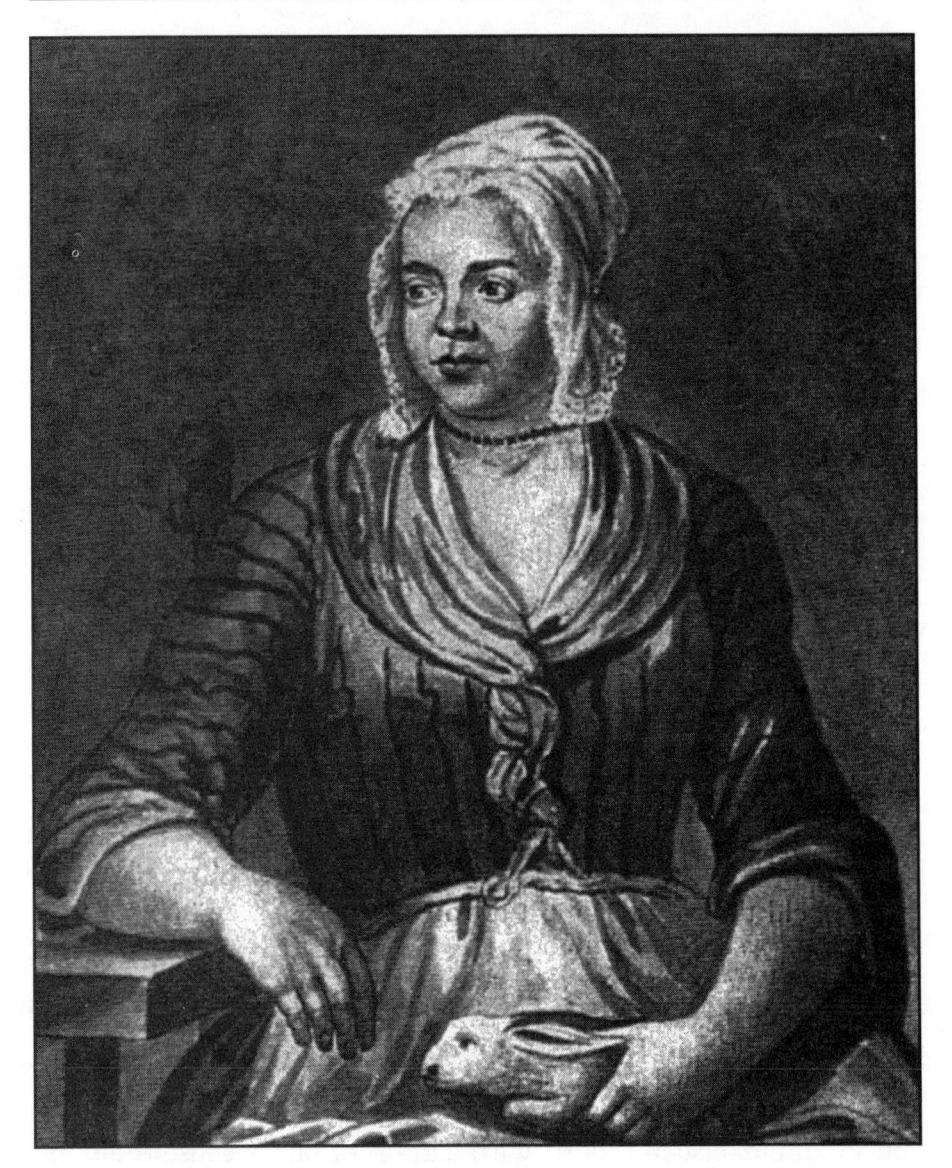

Figure 4. Mary Toft

Painted in 1726 by the artist John Laguerre. From Jan Bondeson, *A Cabinet of Medical Curiosities* (Ithaca, N.Y.: Cornell University Press, 1997), p. 122, fig 1.

from London, said she had a "fair complexion," and "seemed to be of a healthy, strong constituion."[3] In any case, Mary had to have great mental and physical perseverance to survive the hell about to befall her in the hands of medical men and lecherous Londoners. The scrutiny and anger of England would be on her in full force.

Imagine yourself only a few feet away from Mary, watching her as she works in the hop fields, earning a few pennies a day, wishing there were some way out of her poverty. Her back is tired, her hands and feet are sore. The air is filled with the lusty odors of earth and sheep manure. In the distance is the gentle tintinnabulation of cow bells.

Mary's story starts in April 1726 when she was five weeks pregnant. She says she saw a rabbit hop in front of her while she was weeding the garden. She followed it, but it quickly escaped. That night she awakened in a sick fit after dreaming she was in a field with rabbits in her lap. For the next several days, she had an intense desire for rabbit meat—a craving she could not satisfy without the money to buy rabbits at the market. Her desire was so strong that she believed it influenced her reproductive organs. Here is how the 1726 poem "The Doctors in Labour"[4] described it:

When I [Mary Toft] five weeks was gone with
    Child,
And hard at work was weeding in the field,
Up starts a rabbit—to my grief I viewed it,
And vainly though with eagerness pursued it,
The effect was strange—blest is the womb
    that's barren
For that can near be made a coney[5] [rabbit]
    warren.

The rabbit all day long ran in my head,
At night I dreamt I had him in my bed;
Me thought he there a burrow tried to make
His head I patted and stroked his back.
My Husband waked me and cried [Mary] for
    shame
Let go—what was meant I need not name.

In August, Mary suffered a miscarriage. She had abdominal pains and a "large lump of flesh" emerged from her birth canal. Mary described it as "a substance as big as my arm, a truly monstrous birth." Scholars believe her miscarriage was real.[6]

On September 27, Mary had tremendous abdominal pains. She grabbed at her belly and began to shake.

"Get Mary Gill!" Mary Toft yelled.[7] Mary Gill rushed over and found her neighbor writhing in great pain. Mary Gill heard and saw a monstrous birth product fall into a pot between Mary's legs. Mary Gill didn't have the time or stomach to study the baby; however, scientists later inspected the "baby" and found it resembled a liverless cat with the backbone of an eel perched inside its intestines![8]

Mary Gill ran from the house to send for Ann Toft, Mary Toft's mother-in-law and a midwife.

The Toft family gathered around Mary. How could this strange birth happen? Soon, other neighbors came to observe the strange baby. The Tofts decided it was time to consult a medical person of more experience, and they sent the remains of Mary's child to John Howard, Guildford's respected "midwife" and obstetrician. He had been practicing midwifery and surgery for more than thirty years. When Howard studied the monstrous child, he was at first suspicious, then apprehensive. Howard came to the Toft home the next day to see Mary Toft.

"Look at this!" Ann Toft said as she showed Howard some more pieces of a cat that she had taken away from Mary in the night. The neighbors said they witnessed the actual birth.

As Mr. Howard looked between Mary's legs, his sense of horror deepened. Several other parts, perhaps from a pig or cat, came from her womb with the aid of Ann Toft. Howard was unsure of what to make of the astonishing births and so remained the entire day with Mary. Perhaps he suspected a hoax. "I will not be a true believer," he said, "until I deliver something from Mary *myself*." The next day he returned and delivered more cat parts by himself. In spite of this, he was not convinced that the births were genuine. Howard turned to the Tofts. "I'll not be convinced until I deliver the monster's *head*."

There was a relative calm in the Toft house for two weeks, but this was just the eye of the hurricane. In the first week of October, Howard helped Mary deliver a rabbit head while Mary bled profusely.

With the delivery of the head, Howard began to accept her story. It had to be real. And from then on, there was no stopping Mary. Over the next few days, dead rabbit after rabbit came from between her legs. Many times the rabbits were torn into several pieces before leaving her womb. By early November, she was delivering nearly a rabbit a day. Howard gave Mary a little money to help her during these difficult times.

It didn't take long for Howard to become very involved and excited by these miraculous births. Who wouldn't? Imagine yourself called to a neighbor's home to witness monsters falling from a woman in labor. How would you react? Howard wrote enthusiastically about the births to friends, to respected physicians, and to noblemen. Every time Mary delivered, Howard felt bizarre movements in her belly that he attributed to fetal rabbits squirming through her uterus and Fallopian tubes.

Now that Howard had let the cat out of the bag, so to

speak, the entire town became excited by the wondrous births. Huge crowds came to Mary's modest home to see her eerie "children," which Howard preserved and displayed in shiny bottles. After Mary gave birth to her eleventh rabbit carcass, Howard decided it was time to let the entire country know. He offered to present two of her rabbit-babies to England's Royal Society. He wrote to the secretary of King George I:

> As soon as the eleventh rabbit was taken away, up leapt the twelfth rabbit, which is now leaping. If you have any curious person that is please to visit, he may see another leap in her uterus and shall take it from her if he pleases.[9]

Howard had turned from a skeptic into a true believer. One reason for his conversion was the current popular notion that prenatal influences could drastically shape a fetus. He thought Mary's story of craving rabbits played a role in producing strange infants. In addition, Mary's neighbors were convinced that the births were authentic, which helped shape Howard's observations and opinions. And then there were the signs of pregnancy: the bleeding and the powerful abdominal contractions, the snapping sounds from within her womb, and the unpretended pain. Could these be remnants of her August miscarriage? Howard was not sure, but he enjoyed the notoriety he received by being the discoverer of the miraculous births. The fact that he personally delivered rabbits from her vagina and could detect no hoax was probably the biggest factor in his conversion. (Imagine how *you* would feel if you delivered the pieces—would your first thought be of a hoax?) Howard reported:

> When she delivered one rabbit, another was immediately felt in her belly, struggling with such violence that the motion thereof could be sensibly felt and seen: That this motion has sometimes been so strong as to move the bed-clothes, and that it has lasted for twenty and above thirty hours together.[10]

How do you think today's press would handle such a story? Would Mary Toft be on *60 Minutes, Oprah,* or *20/20?* Would the newspapers garble her story? In Mary's time, news of the strange births spread across London, and on October 22, an inaccurate, distorted story was printed in the *British Journal:*

> They write from Guildford that three women working in a field saw a rabbit, which they endeavored to catch, but they could not, they all being with child at the time. One of the women has since, by the help of a man midwife, been delivered of something in the form of a dissected rabbit, with this difference, that one of the legs was like unto a

tabby cat's, and is now kept by the said man Midwife at Guildford.

The amazing births caused quite a royal stir, and even
King George I became intrigued. He immediately ordered
Samuel Molyneux, secretary to the Prince of Wales, to find
out whether the births were authentic or merely some clever
hoax. Court anatomist Nathanael St. André was to accompany Molyneux,[11] who was a clever but amateur scientist and
a fellow of the Royal Society. Molyneux's knowledge of tele-
scopes was great, but of medical matters he knew little.

NOTES

1. King Alfred, also known as Alfred the Great (849–899)
was king of Wessex, a Saxon kingdom in southwestern England.
He prevented England from falling to the Danes and promoted
learning and literacy. Alfred's memory lived on through the Middle
Ages, and in legend, as that of a king who won victory in apparently hopeless circumstances and as a wise lawgiver.

2. Jan Bondeson, *A Cabinet of Medical Curiosities* (Ithaca,
N.Y.: Cornell University Press, 1997), p. 122.

3. Nathanael St. André, *A Short Narrative of an Extraordinary
Delivery of Rabbits, Performed by Mr. John Howard, Surgeon at Guildford* (London, 1727), p. 23.

4. "The Doctor's in Labour; or a New Whim Wham from
Guildford" (London, 1726). This is one of several lyrical celebra-

tions of Mary Toft's story. For readability, I have corrected or modernized the spelling. For example, in the original "rabbet" is often used for "rabbit," "borrough" for "burrow," and so forth.

5. The term "coney" refers to a rabbit, especially the European rabbit (*Oryctolagus cuniculus*). It can also refer to the fur of a rabbit.

6. Dennis Todd, *Imagining Monsters* (Chicago: Chicago University Press, 1995), p. 6.

7. The sequence of events in Mary's story is gleaned from Mary's later confession, several eyewitness accounts, and various scholarly analyses. I have occasionally inserted certain lines of dialogue to convey the story in a dramatic but accurate way. For example, when the literature notes that "Mary sent for her neighbor Mary Gill," I have inserted the dialogue, "Get Mary Gill!" to give the exposition a more immediate feeling. In as much as we may never know the full story because it has been colored through the eyes of various flamboyant personalities, by Mary herself, and by the wisps and eddies of time, dialogue such as this should not unduly obscure the story's veracity and main thrust.

8. Todd, *Imagining Monsters*, pp. 6, 13.

9. Nathanel St. André, *A Short Narrative of an Extraordinary Delivery of Rabbits*, p. 5.

10. Ibid., p. 6.

11. In some accounts, the Prince of Wales asked Samuel Molyneux to investigate, and Molyneux invited Nathanael St. André to accompany him.

CHAPTER TWO

ST. ANDRÉ AND KING GEORGE I

What a chimera, then, is man! What a novelty, what a monster, what a chaos, what a contradiction, what a prodigy! Judge of all things, helpless earthworm, depository of truth, sink of uncertainty and error. Glory and scum of the universe.

—Blaise Pascal, *Pensées*

You have said that the land is a dream for you—and that you fear to be made mad. But madness is not the only danger in dreams. There is also the danger that something may be lost which can never be regained.

—Stephen R. Donaldson, *Lord Foul's Bane*

Things need not have happened to be true. Tales and dreams are the shadow—truths that will endure when mere facts are dust and ashes, and forgot.
—Neil Gaiman, *Neverwhere*

Many myths are based on truth.
—Mr. Spock, "The Way to Eden"

AFTER MARY HAD DELIVERED HER NINTH RABBIT, MIDWIFE John Howard moved Mary Toft from her home in Godalming village to his home at nearby Guildford[1] in Surrey—so it was actually to Guildford that Nathanael St. André and Samuel Molyneux were headed. (Some historians suggest that she did not actually live in Howard's home but in the home of Mrs. Mason, Howard's neighbor.[2]) Howard paid a local woman named Mary Costen to take care of Mary Toft. Mary Toft's sister-in-law, Margaret, also helped out.

Court anatomist Nathanael St. André (figure 5) was one of the most important players in the Mary Toft story and had an unusual past for someone with so distinguished a title. Born in Switzerland, he came with a Jewish family to England as a foot page. Later, he earned a small living teaching German, French, dancing, and fencing. When one of his pupils skewered him, a local surgeon cared for St. André. The surgeon impressed St. André with his wealth and the respect he received from people.

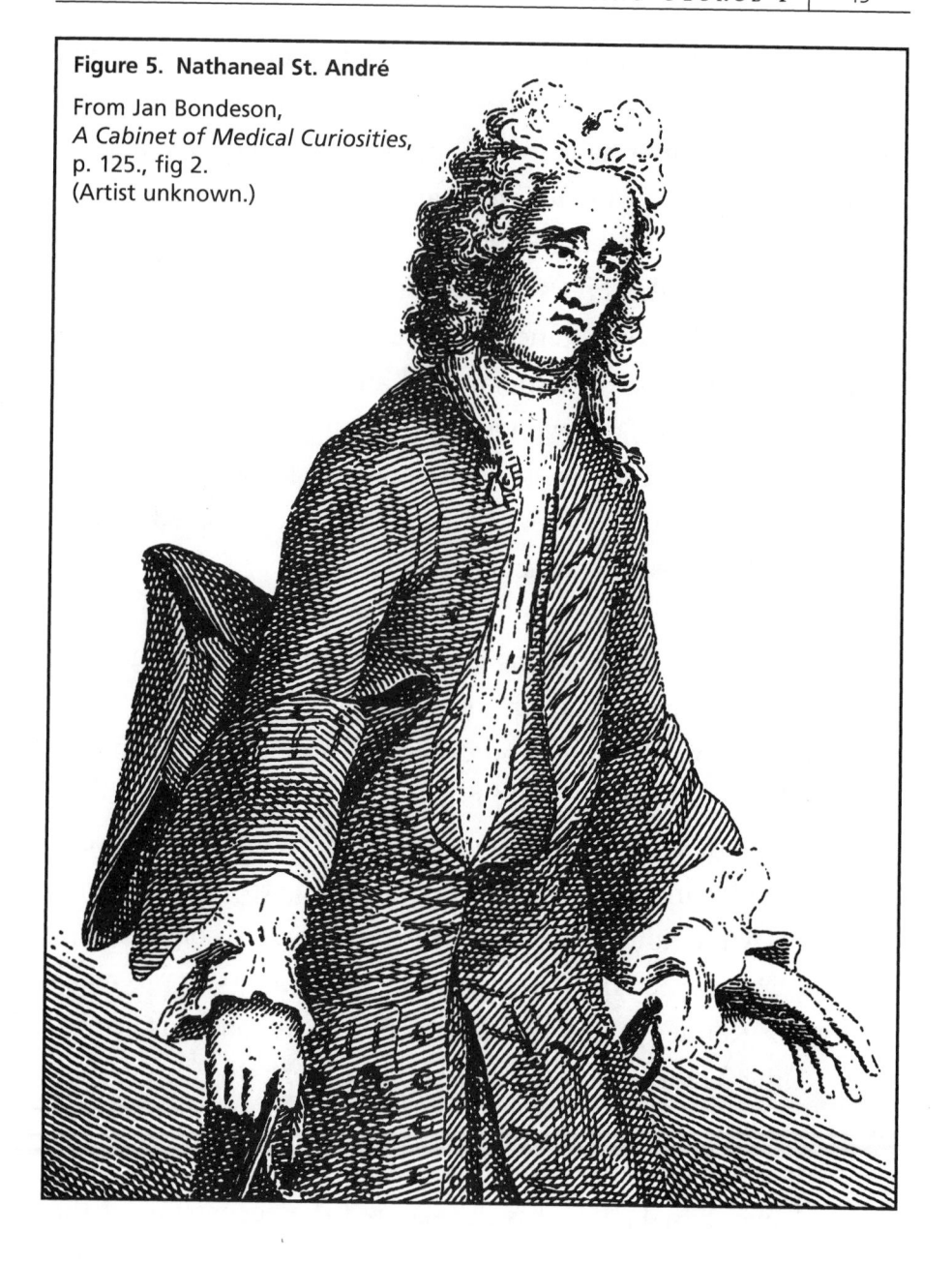

Figure 5. Nathaneal St. André

From Jan Bondeson,
A Cabinet of Medical Curiosities,
p. 125., fig 2.
(Artist unknown.)

From that point on, St. André was determined to be a surgeon. His first step was to become an apprentice to a London surgeon, and after he learned the trade, St. André was able to set up a booming practice while also performing surgery at the Westminster Hospital Dispensary. He never earned a medical degree, but in the 1700s one didn't need a degree to practice medicine. His competency is difficult to ascertain. William Hunter, a famous obstetrician and anatomy teacher, considered St. André "the wonder of his time." Others, such as writer John Nichols, considered St. André a mere "frigid dabbler" in anatomy. Neither opinion seemed to be based on any intimate extensive contact with St. André.

Whatever the case, St. André's German fluency was more helpful to him in becoming court anatomist than his medical prowess. To understand why, we must put Mary Toft's story on hold and consider the mind of King George I for a moment. You'll also get a better feel for the age in which Mary lived by understanding the king's strange court. The odd political climate and goings-on made the public willing to accept strange events while ridiculing the great people involved once deception was suspected. The sex scandals of King George make John F. Kennedy's and Bill Clinton's pale in comparison.

King George I (1660–1727) was born in Osnabrück, Hannover (now in Germany). George succeeded Queen Anne by the terms of the "Act of Settlement," enacted by Parliament in 1701. This act secured the succession of the

English crown to members of the house of Hannover in the Protestant faith.

The transition to King George's reign was peaceful, and "not a mouse stirred against him in England, in Ireland, or in Scotland."[3] Thoroughly German in tastes and habits, King George (figure 6) never learned the English language, and he often returned to Hannover, which always remained his primary concern despite his earnest attempts to attend to England's needs. In fact, George did not rush to England in 1714 when he became king, but rather stopped for festivities and congratulations at several towns in Holland. When he finally arrived two months later, candles and flares were lit as politicians and courtiers jostled to win the favor of their new master (figure 7).

George was rather ambivalent about his powerful new position. He had grown accustomed to the flat north German landscape and his elegant country house, the Herrenhausen, his very own miniature Versailles. Despite this ambivalence, many welcomed the new king with excited verses:

> Hail mighty George! auspicious smiles thy Reign,
> Thee long we wish'd. Thee at last we gain.[4]

The actual attitude of England toward George was probably less jubilant than suggested by the poems and celebrations.

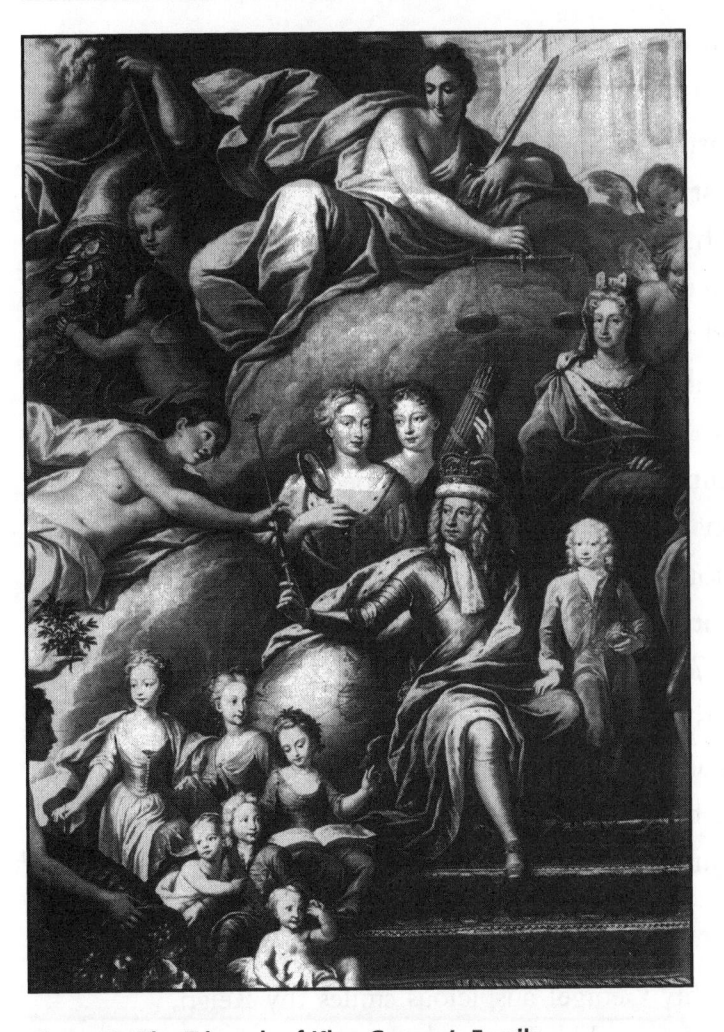

Figure 6. The Triumph of King George's Family

The older woman behind King George I is his mother, Sophia, granddaughter of James I, through whom he inherited the throne. To his right is his daughter Sophia Dorothea and his daughter-in-law Caroline of Anspach (holding the mirror). To his left stands his grandson Frederick, father of George III. His other grandchildren, including William, Duke of Cumberland, are grouped to the left. From Antonia Fraser, *The Lives of the Kings and Queens of England* (Berkeley: University of California Press, 1995), p. 258.

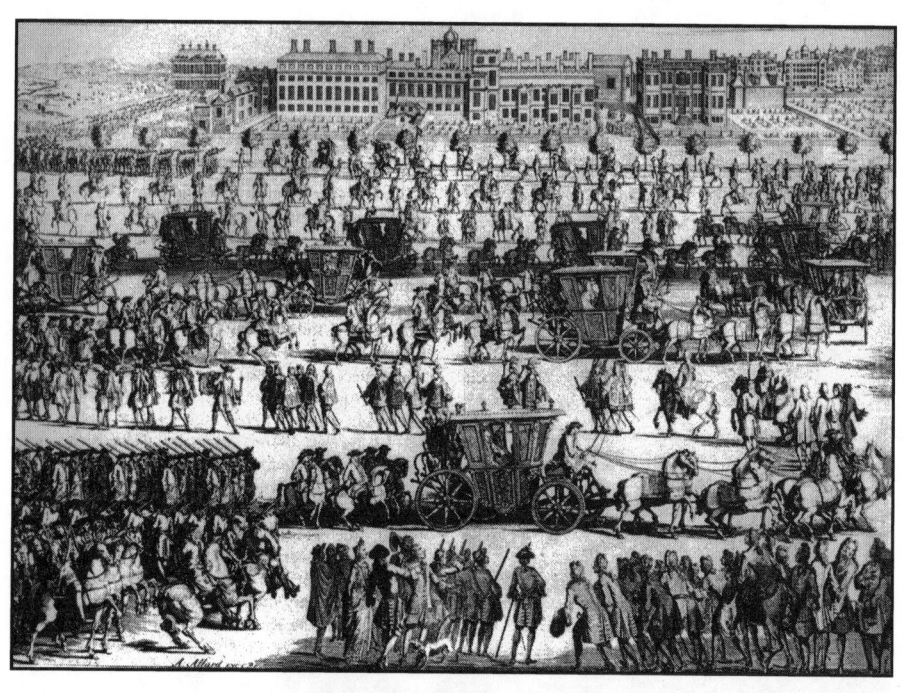

Figure 7. The Coronation Procession of King George I

The procession of George I as it passes St. James's Palace,
his official residence. From Antonia Fraser,
The Lives of the Kings and Queens of England, p. 254.

George's main interests in life were food, horses, and women. He was shy and suspicious but at least he was a good listener. His bravery was unquestionable and everyone knew he had fought hard at the siege of Vienna[5] in 1683.

Despite some of his good qualities, he had a particularly tarnished reputation when it came to marital matters. In 1682, he had married his beautiful cousin Sophia Dorothea of

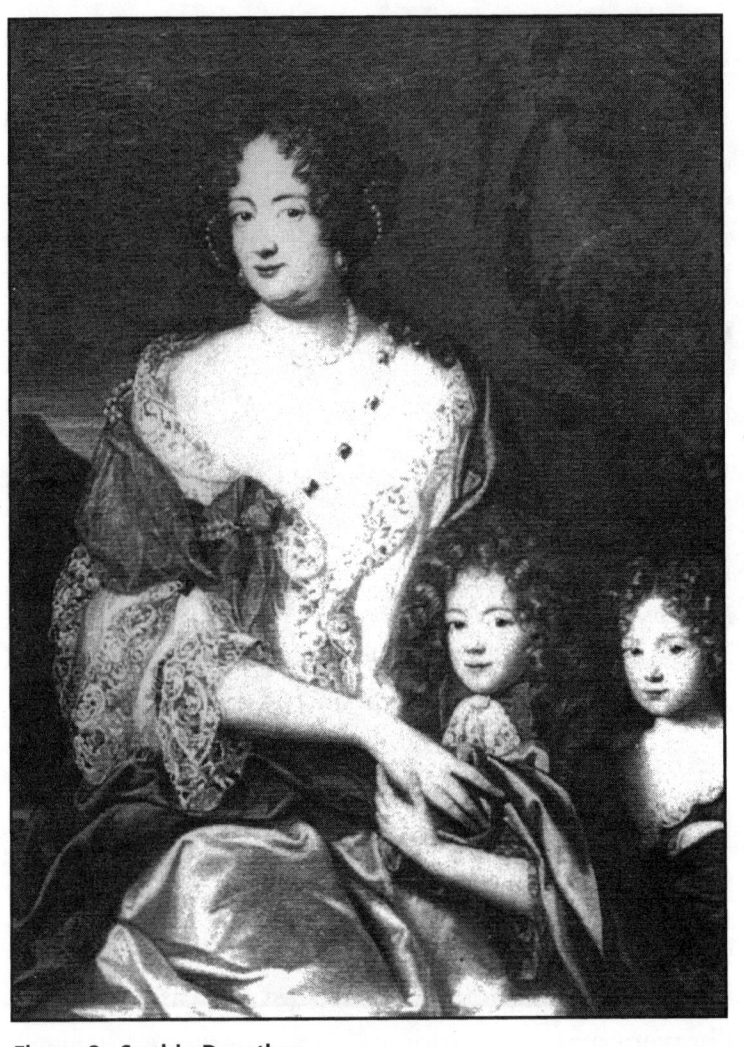

Figure 8. Sophia Dorothea

George's unfortunate wife, Sophia Dorothea, with their two children
George and Sophia Dorothea. When King George discovered her affair
with a Swedish colonel, he confined her to prison at the age of twenty-eight,
where she stayed until she died thirty-two years later. For those thirty-two years,
she was not permitted to see her children. The colonel was hacked to pieces.
From Antonia Fraser, *The Lives of the Kings and Queens of England*, p. 263.

Celle; however, George was a poor husband and paid little attention to Sophia (figure 8). She became bored and developed a passion for Count Philip von Königsmark, a handsome adventurer and Swedish Colonel of Dragoons.[6]

When the colonel started to pay Sophia too much amorous attention, the king had him assassinated—at least that was the rumor. What we do know is that on July 1, 1694, Königsmark disappeared and was never seen again. It is believed that George ordered him hacked to pieces and his mutilated body buried under the floors of Herrenhausen.

King George quickly accused his wife of infidelity, divorced her, and imprisoned her in the castle of Ahlden at the age of twenty-eight where she died thirty-two years later on November 3, 1726, right in the midst of the Mary Toft affair. During those long, lonely years in prison, Sophia Dorothea was never allowed to see her children. On the day King George received the news of his wife's death, he attended a play, and for several months forbid anyone to bury her.

Sophia's son George Augustus was eleven when his mother was imprisoned, and the young boy never forgave his father. After 1714, the Prince of Wales made it clear that he longed for his father's death so Sophia Dorothea might be set free. Hatred dominated the boy's life, and he is alleged to have swam the moat surrounding the Castle at Ahlden in a vain attempt to see his mother.

The public circulated ugly rumors concerning George's

treatment of his wife. To make matters worse, the greed of his two German mistresses did not endear him to the British people. George didn't seem to know how to behave as a real king. He never dined in state but had his meals served in his apartments. His shyness made it hard for him to make new friends, so initially he surrounded himself with only a handful of people who would not make witty jokes about him behind his back. As a result, the court was a strange amalgamation of people like St. André, Turkish servants, and ugly women. One of his German mistresses was unbelievably fat, while the other was as thin as a rail. The super-thin Ehrengard Melusina von Schulenberg (otherwise known as "The Maypole") was nearly sixty. George spent many evenings with her cutting out paper patterns with scissors. The obese Charlotte Sophia Kelmanns (known as "The Castle," who may have been George's half-sister) was more lively than the cadaverous Maypole; however, the Castle's prodigious belly terrified many, including Sir Robert Walpole (1676–1745) when he was a small boy. (Walpole became a British statesman and is generally regarded as the first British prime minister from 1721 to 1742.) Both women grew rich taking bribes from those who wanted royal favors.

Because George spoke almost no English, he communicated with his ministers in French. All George really wanted was to obtain a high position for himself, fill the pockets of his German attendants and mistresses, get away as often as possible from the uncongenial islanders, and use the strength of England to obtain petty advantages for his German principality. Because he had difficulty communicating with his ministers, and because he frequently took trips to Germany, his cabinet had a tendency to assert positions independent from George. Later during his rule, George put his trust in able ministers.

King George's courtiers seemed to enjoy St. André's self-serving, sycophantic behavior, coupled with his command of the German language. In 1723, King George appointed St. André court anatomist, allowing him to treat George for minor maladies.

As much as the king's court liked St. André, some in the medical community despised him. Some of their dislike was born out of jealousy. How could this upstart be appointed so quickly to such a high government position? They called him ignorant, crude, and lecherous. In 1724, He claimed that hired assassins attempted to poison him. St. André may have concocted this hoax to receive sympathy or to make his name more prominent. No culprits were found despite promises of reward. Some of St. André's peers believed he overdosed himself with mercury in an attempt to cure a venereal disease. John Nichols, a contemporary writer, considered the episode "an ostentatious falsehood only to render him an object of attention." Maybe St. André really was attacked. Like several aspects of the Mary Toft story, the entire truth of St. André's own tale is lost in the annals of time.

St. André's name would soon become known throughout England for reasons other than an alleged assassination attempt on his life—namely, his inept handling of Mary Toft. He believed every word she said, until his sad demise. The case would come to national attention in his hands, and his motives, as much as Mary's, would come under close scrutiny.

King George met his own demise a year after the Mary Toft case. In May 1727, George left for Hanover with his beloved "Maypole." A fortuneteller had once told George that he would not outlive his wife by a year. On June 10, 1727, about a year after the Mary Toft miracles, he suffered a paralytic stroke near Osnabrück, Germany, possibly triggered by severe indigestion after binging on melons[7] and suffering the aftereffects of seasickness. He was carried to the Osnabrück castle and died in the very room he had been born. His son George II (1683–1760) ruled Great Britain and Ireland from 1727 to 1760. His daughter Sophia Dorothea (1687–1757) married Frederick William, crown prince (and later king) of Prussia. She was the mother of Frederick the Great.

When news of George's death reached England, there was no national mourning. Newspapers declared, "The Devil has caught him by the throat at last." The king was out of mind so quickly that the English even forgot about burying him. No one thought of returning his body to Westminster Abbey,[8] and George was finally buried at his dearly loved Osnabrück.

Notes

1. Guildford is a town in the county of Surrey, located at the west-east crossing of the River Wey on the north side of the gap by which its valley breaches the chalk ridge of the North Downs.

2. Dennis Todd, *Imagining Monsters* (Chicago: Chicago University Press, 1956), p. 8.

3. Antonia Fraser, *The Lives of the Kings and Queens of England* (Berkeley: University of California Press, 1995), 262.

4. Ibid.

5. The Siege of Vienna (July 17–September 12, 1683) was the Turkish expedition against the Habsburg Holy Roman emperor Leopold I that resulted in their defeat by a combined force led by John III Sobieski of Poland. The siege marked the beginning of the end of Turkish domination in eastern Europe.

6. In early Europe, a dragoon was a mounted soldier who fought as a light cavalryman on attack and as a dismounted infantryman on defense. The term derived from his weapon, a type of carbine or short musket called the dragoon.

7. Karl Shaw, *The Mammoth Book of Tasteless Lists* (New York: Carroll and Graff, 1998), p. 27.

8. Since William the Conqueror, every British sovereign has been crowned in Westminster Abbey except Edward V and Edward VIII, neither of whom was crowned. Many kings and queens are buried near the shrine of Edward the Confessor or in Henry VII's chapel. The last sovereign to be buried in the abbey was George II (d. 1760); since then they have been buried at Windsor.

CHAPTER THREE

RABBIT DUNG

I have always been intrigued by fringe science, perhaps for the same reason that I enjoy freak shows at carnivals and circuses. Pseudoscientists, especially the extreme cranks, are fascinating creatures for psychological study. Moreover, I have found that one of the best ways to learn something about any branch of science is to find out where its crackpots go wrong.

—Martin Gardner, *On the Wild Side*

What crime is greater than that of deliberately mistreating the public about science, of deliberately misleading them, of defrauding them, of feeding and stimulating their ignorance?
—Isaac Asimov, *I. Asimov*

And if a woman approach unto any beast, and lie down thereto, thou shalt kill the woman, and the beast: they shall surely be put to death; their blood [shall be] upon them.
—Leviticus 20:16

Sex: the pleasure is momentary, the position ridiculous, and the expense damnable.
—Lord Chesterfield (1694–1773)

MARY TOFT'S EIGHTEENTH CENTURY IS SOMETIMES called the "Age of Enlightenment." It opened with the War of Spanish Succession[1] and closed with the French Revolution.[2] In between it saw the birth of the United States, which had withdrawn from England to create its own constitution in 1787. It was a century of political disruption and revolutionary idealism that extended to all fields of thought.[3]

In scientific areas, eighteenth-century Europeans slowly began to accept only what was observable directly and reproducible by experiment. This was a result of increasing respect for the experimental method, which was the foundation of research since Galileo Galilei (1564–1642), the Italian mathematician, astronomer, and physicist. As the first man to use the telescope to study the skies, Galileo proved the Earth revolves around the Sun and was not the center of the universe. By the eighteenth century, the teaching of anatomy was fully established in the medical schools of Europe.

The eighteenth century also saw the rise of physicians who based their practice on scientific knowledge. The best doctors of the period, like the Dutchman Hermann Boerhaave (1668–1738), were among the finest clinicians of all time. Others like the Frenchman Philippe Pinel (1745–1826) pioneered the humane treatment of the mentally ill so that, for the first time, the insane were treated as other sick people rather than locked in prisons with dangerous criminals.

Despite these advances, the eighteenth century was also the heyday of charlatans and mystics. For example, the German doctor Ernst Stahl (1660–1734) promoted "animism," which said that illness was the soul's healing effort to get rid of morbid matter from the body. Illness was the tendency of the soul to reestablish order in bodily functions. The ideas of Franz Anton Mesmer (1734–1815) also grew in popularity. Mesmer was the German physician whose system of therapeutics, known as mesmerism, was the forerunner of the modern practice of hypnotism. Mesmer suggested that planets' gravitational attraction affected human health by interacting with an invisible fluid found in the human body and throughout

nature. In 1775, Mesmer revised his theory of "animal gravita-
tion" to one of "animal magnetism," wherein the body's invisible fluid acted according to the laws of magnetism. According
to Mesmer, "animal magnetism" could be activated by any
magnetized object and manipulated by a trained person. Disease resulted from "obstacles" in the fluid's flow through the
body, and these obstacles could be broken by "crises" (trance
states often ending in delirium or convulsions). Mesmer
devised various therapeutic treatments to achieve harmonious
fluid flow, and in many of these treatments he was a forceful
and rather dramatic personal participant.

Obstetrics had become a branch of medicine in the seventeenth century, when midwives were relegated to secondary
place as surgeons and physicians began to compete for
supremacy in this field. The first specialists appeared in the
eighteenth century and began to make thorough studies of the
female reproductive organs, particularly during pregnancy.

In short, Mary Toft lived in a time when science, literature,
and culture were advancing at a fast rate. The year Mary had
her rabbits, Jonathan Swift published *Gulliver's Travels*, and
Stephen Hales accurately measured blood pressure. It was also
the decade when Johann Sebastian Bach's "Brandeburg Con-
certos" and Georg Frideric Handel's "Water Music" stirred our
hearts, and the Quakers were demanding abolition of slavery.
Inoculation against smallpox was introduced in England five
years before Mary had her rabbits, Isaac Newton's great *Prin-*

cipia was translated three years after, and Benjamin Franklin issued his *Poor Richard's Almanac* six years later.

Given the state of science and medicine, most medical men of Mary's time *should* have suspected that humans cannot give birth to rabbits! This is not to say that the eighteenth-century people didn't have some peculiar ideas by today's standards. One of the early eighteenth-century English folk cures for mumps was to lead the patient three times around a pigsty while in the halter of an ass. In Edinburgh the writer and lecturer John Brown suggested that there were only two diseases, stenthia (strong) and asthenia (weak), and two treatments, stimulant and sedative; his remedies were alcohol and opium. Passionate debate took place between his followers, the Brunonians, and the more orthodox Cullenians (followers of William Cullen, a professor of medicine at Glasgow). The controversy over how to best treat diseases spread to the medical centers of Europe.

Also during the eighteenth century, Samuel Hahnemann of Leipzig originated homeopathy, a treatment system in which he administered minute doses of drugs. The drugs' effects resembled the effects of the disease being treated. In some ways, his odd ideas had an unintended positive effect upon medicine at a time when prescriptions were lengthy and doses were large.

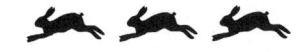

In eighteenth-century London, Scottish doctors were the leaders in surgery and obstetrics.[4] The famous teacher John Hunter conducted important research in comparative anatomy and physiology, founded surgical pathology, and raised surgery to the level of a respectable branch of science. His brother William Hunter, an eminent anatomy teacher, became famous as an obstetrician. Male doctors were now attending women in childbirth. About thirty years after Mary Toft gave birth, British obstetrician William Smellie's *Treatise on the Theory and Practice of Midwifery* contained the first systematic discussion on the safe use of obstetrical forceps, which have since saved countless lives. Smellie placed midwifery on a sound scientific footing and helped to establish obstetrics as a recognized medical discipline. (One wonders how the Mary Toft story would have played out if Dr. Smellie had been present at her strange deliveries.)

The science of modern pathology also had its beginnings in the 1700s. In 1761, Giovanni Battista Morgagni of Padua published his massive work *De Sedibus et Causis Morborum* (The seats and causes of diseases investigated by anatomy), a description of 700 postmortem examinations in which he correlated afterdeath findings with the clinical picture in life.

One very important medical advance, late in the century, was vaccination. Smallpox had often been disfiguring and fatal.

Inoculation had been practiced in the East, and then popular-
ized in England in 1721–22 by Lady Mary Wortley Montagu.
She had observed the practice in Turkey, where it produced a
mild form of the disease and then gave immunity to the person.
It was not until 1796 that Edward Jenner, a country practitioner
and John Hunter's pupil, began inoculations with cowpox (the
bovine form of the disease). When he later inoculated the same
subject with smallpox, the disease did not appear.

Many old-fashioned ways were being tossed aside in the
eighteenth century. As we mentioned, in Paris, Philippe Pinel
initiated bold reforms in the care of the mentally ill, releasing
them from their chains and discarding the long-held notion
that insanity was caused by demon possession. James Lind, a
British naval surgeon from Edinburgh, recommended fresh
fruits and citrus juices to prevent scurvy. In 1752, John
Pringle, a Scotsman, published his *Observations on the Diseases
of the Army*, which contained numerous recommendations for
the troops' health and comfort. He had served with the
British forces during the War of the Austrian Succession, and
he suggested in 1743 that military hospitals on both sides
should be regarded as sanctuaries; this plan eventually led to
the establishment of the Red Cross organization in 1864.

Clear scientific thinking was making steady progress, and
advances in physics, chemistry, and the biological sciences
were converging to form a rational scientific basis for every
branch of clinical medicine. New knowledge spread through-

out Europe and traveled across the sea, where centers of medical excellence were being established in America.

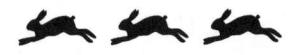

With this introduction to medicine in the 1700s, let us return to our story where we last left court surgeon St. André and Royal Society Fellow Samuel Molyneux riding to Guildford to examine Mary Toft. When they arrived at John Howard's home on November 15, Howard came rushing out to greet them.

"Sirs," Howard said, "Come quickly. Mary Toft is in labor with her fifteenth rabbit!"

St. André went inside and approached Mary who was surrounded by women attendants. In just a few minutes, he delivered from her a skinned rabbit that appeared to be about four months old (figure 9). Inside were the heart, diaphragm, and lungs.

"If we study the lungs," St. André said to Molyneux, "we may obtain some clue about the rabbit's true origin."

Molyneux nodded as they plopped the wet lungs into a jar of water and noticed that they floated. St. André later wrote:

> I instantly cut off a piece of lungs and tried them in water; they seemed but just specifically lighter than it, and Mr. Molyneux pressing them to the bottom found they rose again very slowly.

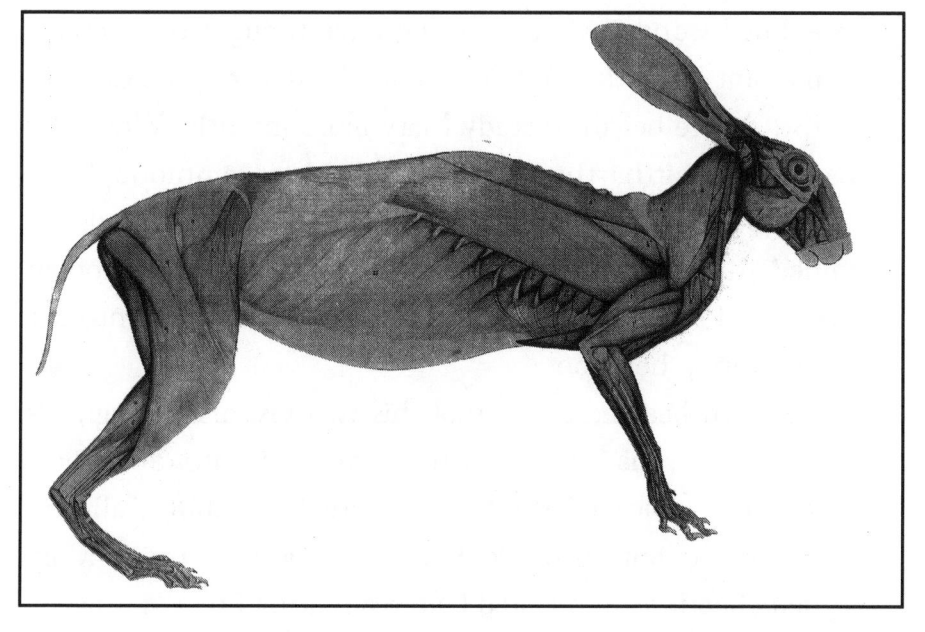

Figure 9. The Hare

This anatomical drawing shows the musculature of a hare.
From W. Ellenberger, H. Dittrich, and H. Baum,
An Atlas of Animal History (New York: Dover, 1956), p. 140.

In hindsight, you and I might think that *floating* lungs proved that the rabbit had actually breathed air before it died, and therefore could not have developed inside Mary's uterus, but St. André concluded that the "preternatural" rabbit did not follow the known laws of physics. In any case, St. André said that the lungs were smaller and darker than the lungs of rabbits that had breathed for some time. (Isaac Newton died the next year and may not have actively followed Mary Toft's tale, but I wonder what he would have thought of supernatural rabbit lungs that did not follow the laws of physics.)

St. André began to study Mary more intently. When she had given birth, there was no blood or amniotic fluid, although he was able to get milk from her breasts. He determined that there were some "inequalities" in her fallopian tubes, and that the rabbits, bred in the tubes, came into her uterus during her labor.

Howard beamed as he took his two visitors through his home, which had been partly converted into a medical museum that housed the fourteen previous rabbits, all preserved in big bottles of alcohol. From the next room, Mary sighed cheerfully and rested before a roaring fire.

St. André and Molyneux stooped down to examine Howard's gruesome collection of gray and pink masses floating in liquid. They noticed that the first specimen had cat's paws, but that all the others resembled few-month-old rabbits. All of the creatures had been delivered in pieces.

"I believe," said Mr. Howard, "that the creatures were torn to pieces by Mary's strong uterine contractions."

When St. André took some pieces out of the jar to examine them more closely, he found nothing particularly notable about Mary Toft's babies, except, of course, that they were not human.

"Somethin's coming!" Mary moaned from the nearby room.

While the men had been studying Mary's children, Mary Toft had started going into labor again, within two hours of her previous delivery. They rushed back to her room.

"What is it?" Howard said.

"I do not know," Mary said, and within minutes out came the lower portion of a male rabbit. Again, the rabbit had no skin. This time the part fit perfectly with the portion delivered earlier that day.

When St. André and Molyneux dissected this bottom carcass, they found several pellets in the rectum. St. André examined the creature's rectum:

> In the rectum we found five or six pellets, much of the same colour and consistence as the common dung of a rabbit, little bodies, like dried fragments, being matted together with a mucous matter.

Rather than considering the "common" dung as evidence that the rabbit did not develop inside Mary's womb, St. André again took this as evidence of supernatural, or as he put it, "preternatural" happenings.

One by one, St. André carefully opened the intestines of Mary's previous rabbit-children and found in some only mucous like that found in fetal animals. When he cut open the intestine of Mary Toft's first monster, St. André discovered what appeared to be the bones of an eel.

Later in the night, Mary fell again into a wild labor. It took five people to hold her down and stop her from flailing about.

"Wait!" St. André said. "Let me check you before anything else happens." He reached into her vagina and found it to be clear. Her cervix was closed. He watched her closely, did not let anyone else get near her, and after several minutes, he delivered some fur all rolled up in a ball. St. André claimed that he kept his hand in her vagina the whole time to eliminate the possibility of fraud.

There was a shriek from Mary. Ten minutes later came a rabbit head with the fur still attached. One ear was missing.

St. André was excited and began to examine her abdomen. He thought he felt some irregularity with one of her ovaries. He also felt the weird pulsations that John Howard had noticed earlier. "The movements," Howard said, "are caused by tiny rabbits jumping within Mary's Fallopian tubes."

St. André didn't want to leave all the physical evidence behind in Guildford, and insisted on taking rabbit specimens back to London to show King George and the Prince of Wales. The next day, in London, Molyneux and St. André together dissected Mary's babies so that they could compare them to ordinary rabbits. The results were inconclusive. Here is a summary of St. André's findings:

- Bodies—large, the size of two- to four-month old rabbits.

- Lungs—cannot tell if they had breathed air; smaller than newborn rabbit lungs.
- Hearts—comparatively bulky. Each heart contains an open foramen ovale, suggesting the rabbits are fetuses.*
- Liver—comparatively bulky.
- Intestines—smaller than newborns' intestines. Some contain pellets like those of rabbits who feed outside the womb, while other intestines contain fetal mucous. In the first monster Mary birthed, there are fragments of an eel bone. Most of the monster's parts resemble those of a cat. No explanation for this anomaly.
- Bones—appear to have fetal characteristics.
- Teeth—not worn.

Although these results were contradictory and the observations inexact, St. André convinced himself that these were signs of a preternatural creature with "the strongest marks of fetuses, even by such parts that cannot exist in an adult." He went on to write, "This, I think, proves in the strongest terms possible that these animals were of a particular kind, and *not* bred in a natural way." He did not suspect fraud. He had watched Mary carefully during her deliveries and saw no signs of foul play.

Perhaps King George had a sneaking doubt about the

---

*An opening in the heart wall is normal before birth, but it usually closes at birth or shortly thereafter.

whole affair. We do not know for sure. We do know that Mary Toft's story spread through London like wildfire. King George asked Cyriacus Ahlers, a German surgeon, to investigate further. Ahlers and his friend Mr. Brand, who was related to the king's apothecary, arrived in Guildford on Sunday morning, November 20.

From the very start Ahlers was a skeptic; however, he initially kept his skepticism to himself. Ahlers reasoned that if he *appeared* to believe Mary's story he might be able to more easily discover a hoax.

Mr. Howard brought Ahlers and Mr. Brand to Mary Toft where a nurse told them that Mary had just delivered a rabbit skin. Ahlers studied the skin and found very little blood or fluid. Mary did not appear pregnant: her stomach was not swollen, and her breasts gave no milk. His suspicions intensified when he found her pulse to be normal and when she walked into the room holding her thighs close together, as if "she were afraid something might drop down, which she did not care to lose." Not only did Ahlers suspect Mary, he also considered Mr. Howard a collaborator in an elaborate fraud.

Mary started to go into labor. "It's coming!"

"Reach into her," Mr. Howard said to Ahlers. "What do you feel?"

Mr. Howard placed his fingers inside Mary's vagina and felt broken bones and some flesh protruding from the vagina. It appeared to be the back end of a rabbit.

Ahlers turned to Mr. Howard. "Why are all the rabbits coming from Mary skinned?"

Mr. Howard nodded. "It is her womb's unnaturally strong convulsive motions. They rub the rabbits against Mary's pubic bone and remove the skin."

Ahlers pretended to accept this explanation as Mary roared and screamed throughout the delivery. When Ahlers asked Mr. Howard how Mary could laugh during her delivery at their occasional jokes, Mr. Howard suggested it was her strong body and will.

Unfortunately, Ahlers was not an obstetrician and he hurt Mary while trying to remove the back end of the rabbit. In fact, he accidentally pushed it in further, which caused her horrific discomfort. Seeing Ahlers fumble and put Mary in great pain, Howard refused to let Ahlers deliver another rabbit. This caused Ahlers to be even more suspicious of fraud.

"You're hurting her," Mr. Howard said. "*I* will do it." He then delivered the forepart of the rabbit.

To throw Mr. Howard and Mary off track, Ahlers appeared to accept the whole birthing scenario. He told Howard, "I am *fully* satisfied, and convinced of the truth, and can have no doubts after such proofs." He pretended to have compassion for Mary and promised to ask the king to give her a pension.

Ahlers gazed at the rabbit parts. "May I bring the pieces back to London?"

Howard nodded. "But you must promise to return me the parts."

"Certainly," said Ahlers as he gave Mary some money, collected the various rabbit parts (except for some of the intestines that had gotten trampled on the floor), and began examining the intestines he had left. In the rectum of one rabbit were pellets of hard dung. Howard removed them with a sharp pin and put them in a pretty box for Ahlers to take with him.

Back in London, Ahlers began a more leisurely study of the creatures. He believed that the rabbit bones and muscles were clearly cut with a knife and could not have been torn apart simply by Mary's uterine contractions. The dung contained hay, straw, and corn. In Ahlers' mind there was no doubt that Mary Toft and Howard were perpetrating a hoax. On Monday, November 21, Ahlers reported on his investigation to King George. Ahler's began to tell members of the court that he strongly suspected a hoax, and he also showed the rabbit specimens as evidence.

News of Ahlers' suspicions spread fast. To make a strong case for himself and to discredit Ahlers, on November 22, Howard wrote an open letter to the newspapers saying that Ahlers had told *everyone* in Guildford that the rabbit births were *genuine*.

On Wednesday, November 23, realizing that his own reputation was at stake, St. André rushed back to Guildford with his friend Mr. D'Anteney, a polymath interested in mechanics, geometry, and cryptography. Mary Toft proceeded to deliver membranes that Howard and St. André thought were parts of the chorion, the outermost membrane around the embryo. Could it have been a *human* chorion? They never could tell for sure. In mammals (except marsupials), the chorion develops a rich blood vessel supply and is associated with the uterus's endometrium (lining). Chorion and endometrium together form the placenta, which is the embryo's principal organ of respiration, nutrition, and excretion.

Placing the "chorion" aside, St. André and Howard made sure that the public believed Ahlers to be a hypocrite, someone who assured all the people in Guildford that the births were genuine, someone who gave Mary money and said he would help her get a pension from the king.

The press had a field day interviewing the people in Guildford. Elizabeth Helmes, owner of the nearby White Hart Inn, said, "Ahlers assured me he would convince all the unbelievers when he returned to London!" Mary Costen, Mary Toft's nurse, told the press, "Ahlers declared it was wonderful people would not believe a fact that was so true as this appeared to him." Howard's brother Thomas said, "Ahlers was *convinced* the rabbits had come from Mary's uterus."

In summary, St. André and the people of Guildford wanted to know if Ahlers had lied to them, how could he be trusted now? They said Ahlers' skepticism was insincere and unfair. His investigation was shallow and incomplete. Almost all of St. André's arguments dealt with Ahlers' character, and not the scientific evidence. As would become clear in the coming days, the Mary Toft case would not be relegated to mere scientific investigation but to public accusations against all personalities involved.

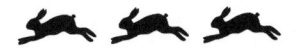

On November 25, St. André started to write a detailed account of his observations entitled *A Short Narrative of an Extraordinary Delivery of Rabbits*, to which Molyneux added a scientific-sounding postscript stating that the deliveries did not appear to be a hoax. In this document, St. André openly challenged Ahlers. Anticipating further rabbit births, St. André quickly added that "*The Account of the Delivery of the Eighteenth Rabbit* shall be published by way of an Appendix to his account."

On November 26, St. André further dissected the first, third, fifth, and ninth rabbits in front of a huge audience consisting of King George, the Prince of Wales, and members of the nobility. The upper-class audience seemed convinced that St. André had evidence of real rabbit births. St. André enjoyed being in the public eye and was willing to use various tactics of self-promotion. In the past he had placed advertisements in London newspapers announcing his court appointment and promoting his skills. When he had been allegedly poisoned by assassins, he gave a detailed daily record of his heroic struggle against death, and publicized his relationships with the court and king.

Meanwhile, St. André's pamphlet *A Short Narrative of an Extraordinary Delivery of Rabbits* promptly became a bestseller! The whole country was gossiping about Mary Toft.

Lord John Hervey—an English politician whose *Memoirs of the Reign of George the Second* are largely responsible for our impressions of eighteenth-century England—wrote the following to politician Henry Fox:

> There is a thing that employs everybody's tongue at present, which is a woman brought out of Surrey who has brought forth seventeen rabbits, and has been there these days in labour of the eighteenth. I know you laugh now, and this I joke; but the fact as reported and attested by St. André the surgeon (who swears he has delivered her of five) is something that really staggers one.

Londoners debated whether the story was true, and St. André invited many distinguished people to visit Mary and her strange children. Some religious people suspected witchcraft and suggested that Mary was actually a rabbit who had metamorphosed into a human. (Luckily, the last execution for witchcraft in England was in 1712.)

The rumors, speculations, and innuendoes were endless. A few people claimed Mary had sex with rabbits, which led to her rabbit babies. One of the local writers theorized that Mary kept a large buck rabbit in her home and performed various unspecified "acts of kindness." Others suggested that Mary had stuffed a pregnant female rabbit within her uterus! The rabbit would periodically give birth, and the babies would shoot out Mary's vagina.

NOTES

1. The War of Spanish Succession (1701–14) arose out of the disputed succession to the Spanish throne following the death of the childless Charles II, the last of the Spanish Habsburgs

2. The French Revolution shook France between 1787 and 1799, and reached its first climax there in 1789.

3. Roberto Margotta, *The Story of Medicine* (New York: Golden Press, 1968), p. 221.

4. "Medicine: The History of Medicine and Surgery: Medicine and Surgery before 1800: The Enlightenment: Medicine in the Eighteenth Century," *Britannica Online* (http://www.eb.com).

CHAPTER FOUR

WHY ANIMALS
AND SEX?

The broad mass of a nation will more easily fall victim to a big lie than to a small one.

— Adolph Hitler, *Mein Kampf*

There are no such things as lies, only truths looking for new premises.

— Wolf Gort, *A Life of Deceit*

Never lie when the truth is more profitable.

— Stanislaw J. Lec

> *All great truths begin as blasphemies.*
> —George Bernard Shaw, *Anajanska*

> *I am brother to dragons, and a companion to owls.*
> —Job 30:29

THIS CHAPTER WILL AMAZE SOME AND DISGUST OTHERS. However, I want to place our discussion of animal births and beliefs in perspective with both Mary's time and human civilizations in general. Those with weak stomachs may skip the bizarre extravaganza that follows.

All of the crazy speculation about Mary's births would seem silly, unbelievable, or totally out of place to us today if we weren't constantly barraged with tabloid headlines like "Woman Gives Birth to Alligator Child" or "Woman Gives Birth to Duck Boy." For your edification and intellectual stimulation, here are some recent sample headlines from the *Weekly World News*:[1]

- Bat Child Found in Cave!
- Half-Human Half-Fish Found in Florida!
- Bat with Human Face!
- Hillary Clinton Adopts Alien Baby!
- *Titanic* Baby Found Alive!
- X-Rays Reveal Baby's Head on Backward! Doctors will operate to set boy's head straight!

Of course, most people probably laugh at these titles, not taking them seriously. Yet, notice how many titles deal with our incessant preoccupation with strange births of animal-like creatures. Perhaps they capitalize on our subliminal fears. In some ways, little has changed since the time of Mary Toft. Today the Internet spreads numerous urban legends involving animals and strange births.

Our fascination with animals starts at childhood with fairy tales and myths. Ever wonder why children's stories have animal protagonists? The best answer is that the animals, though childlike, are slightly different from real children, and this makes the dramatic events of fairy tales, scary bedtime stories, and TV cartoons a little easier to handle.[2] The basic fairy tale confronts a fear in the child's life—getting lost, getting into trouble, dealing with wickedness or poverty—and shows how such events can be triumphed. The use of animals allows the child to empathize with the characters but maintain sufficient distance to dampen the mental anguish. Many psychologists suggest that children require the disguise or symbolism of animals to talk about their feelings.

Some of Mary's contemporaries believed Mary actually cavorted with rabbits—but this is not as odd as it might seem. Through the ages, men and women have had sexual relations with a wide variety of animals, such as domestic pets, although rarely for the purposes of procreation. Roman women used the heads of live snakes for stimulation.[3] At other times, women have placed the tails of live fishes into their vaginas, or smeared honey on the vulva to attract flies; "the flies thus attracted by the honey would tickle the woman until her sexual appetite was appeased."[4]

In pre-Mao-Zedong China, a significant number of men enjoyed copulating with geese.[5] At the moment of ejaculation, the man would pull the head of the live animal to get "the pleasurable benefit of the anal sphincter's last spasms in the victim."[6] Marquis De Sade (1740–1814)—the French nobleman whose perverse sexual preferences gave rise to the term sadism—commented that turkeys were used in Parisian brothels, where the act was termed aviosodomy.

Men and women have copulated with a wide variety of animals to demonstrate piety and religions devotion. (For a complete accounting of "religions bestiality" involving camels, cattle, monkeys and baboons, you should read the works of G. L. Simons.[7]) Bestiality was also a common form of entertainment in the Roman arena where mass public displays of bestiality were "a phenomenon unique in history."[8] Beasts were specially trained to copulate with women; if the girls or women were unwilling, then the animal would attempt rape. An astonishing array of creatures were used for these practices—bulls, donkeys, giraffes, leopards, zebras, stallions, large dogs, apes, cheetahs.

In 1933, writer Gaston Dubois-Desauule discussed many allegedly true cases of animals being born to woman.[9] For example, Catholic inquisitor Martin Del Rio claimed that women "have been seen to give birth to a dormouse, another to a savage rat, and another to a monster resembling a bear." Torquemada (1420–1498), the brutal Spanish Inquisitor, believed that these animal births were punishments God gave to women who "gave themselves to disordered and abominable couplings."

Perhaps the strong public interest in Mary Toft was also a reflection of lingering horror and fascination with animals which were everywhere in sixteenth-century witch trials. For example, witches were sometimes forced to confess they had had children by the devil, who often took the form of a goat (an image that lingered into the nineteenth century; see figure 10). In the year 1561, five poor women of Verneuil, France, were accused of transforming themselves into cats in front of Satan who presided over them in goat form. They were found guilty and burned alive. In 1564, while being tortured, four people admitted they saw a great black goat that spoke to them and made them kiss him. The four were executed at Poitiers. In 1573, at Dôle, France, Gilles Garnier was indicted for being a *loup-garour* or man-wolf and for prowling in that shape at night to devour little children (figure 11). He was burned alive for his admissions coerced through torture on the rack.[10]

The close proximity of bestiality and witchcraft accusations is evident when Françoise Sécretain was burned alive

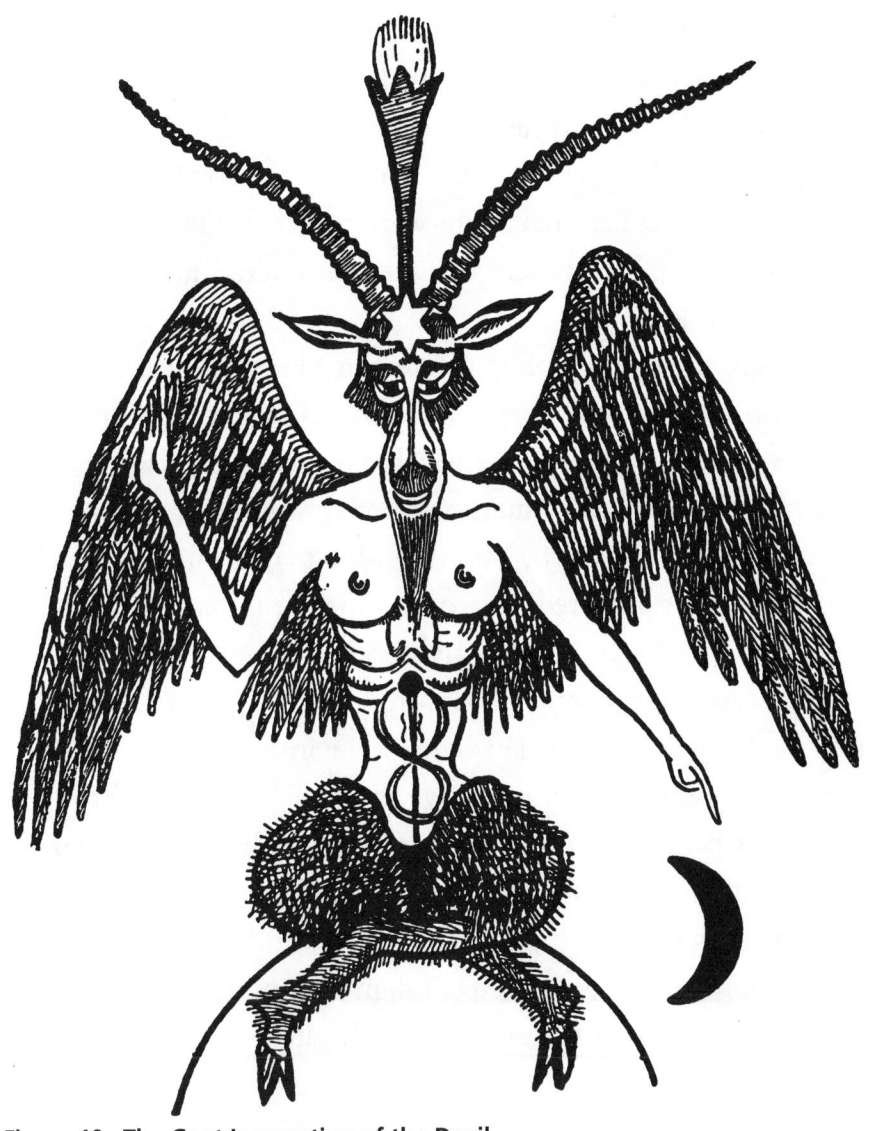

Figure 10. The Goat Incarnation of the Devil

From Ernst Lehner and Johanna Lehner, *Picture Book of Devils, Demons, and Witchcraft* (New York: Dover, 1971), p. 22, fig. 49. After Eliphas Levi, from a pen drawing in a French occult manuscript *La Magie Noire* (Black Magic), nineteenth century.

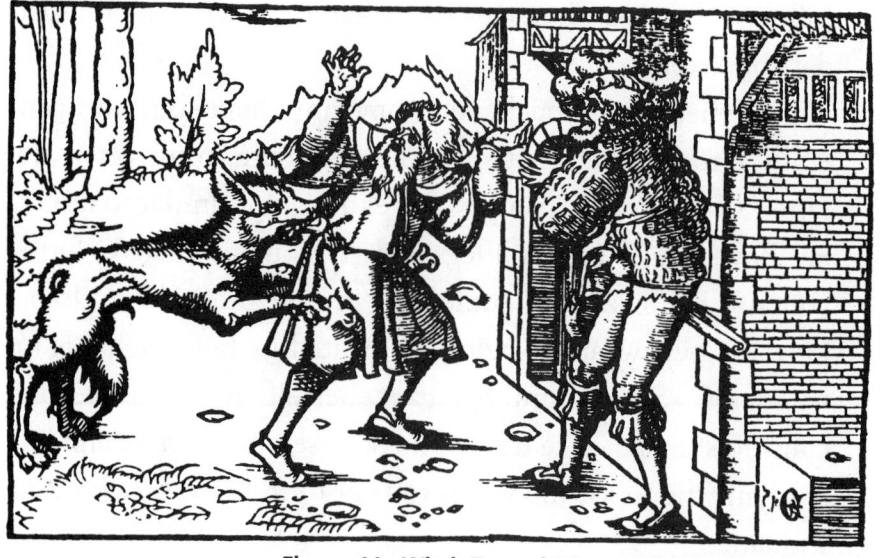

Figure 11. Witch Turned Werewolf Attacking Travelers

From Ernst Lehner and Johanna Lehner,
Picture Book of Devils, Demons, and Witchcraft, p. 64, fig. 91.
Woodcut by Hans Weiditz, from Dr. Johann Geiler von Kayserberg,
Die Emies (The Ants), printed by Johann Grüninger, Strassburg, 1517.

because she had had carnal knowledge of domestic animals—a dog, a cat, and a cock—and because she admitted she was a witch and her animals were earthly forms of the devil.[11] Another case of theriomorphism (animal forms representing the divine or supernatural) occurred in 1474, when Basle magistrates sentenced a cock to be burned at the stake "for the heinous and unnatural crime of laying an egg." It was widely believed that the oeuf coquatri (egg material) was the main ingredient in witch ointment and, when the egg was hatched by a snake or a toad, monsters such as basilisks would hide in a house and destroy the inhabitants with their death-darting eyes.

Witches were thought to assume any shape, but they generally chose either that of a cat or a hare, most often the latter. (Technically speaking, hares are quite similar to rabbits but have longer ears and legs and give birth to active, furred young.) For example, sometime in the late 1590s, Isabel Gowdie grew weary of being persecuted by her neighbors for witchcraft. She voluntarily gave herself up to justice and claimed she had once transformed herself into a hare and had to chant the following words to transform herself back into a woman:

> Hare! hare!
> God send thee care!
> I am in hare's likeness now;
> But I shall be a woman e'en now!
> Hare! hare!
> God send thee care![12]

The sixteenth-century witch hunts are among the best (and saddest) examples of the dangers of irrational thinking. One contemporary critic of the witch craze, Johann Matthäus Meyfarth, wrote that he would give all his money away if he could banish the memory of what the pious did to many thousands of helpless women to elicit confessions:

I have seen the limbs forced asunder, the eyes
driven out of the head, the feet torn from the legs,
the sinews twisted from the joints, the shoulder
blades wrung from their place, the deep veins
swollen, the superficial veins driven in, the victim
hoisted aloft and now dropped, now revolved
around, head undermost and feet uppermost. I have
seen the executioner flog with the scourge, and
smite with rods, and crush with screws, and load
down with weights, and stick with needles, and
bind around with cords, and burn with brimstone,
and baste with oil and singe with torches. In short,
I can bear witness, I can describe, I can deplore how
the human body is violated.[13]

Matthew Hopkins, a seventeenth-century witch-finder,
had some of the strangest ideas about women and their relations with animals. While in England, he would place a suspected witch in the middle of a room upon a stool or table in
some uneasy posture. If she refused to sit in this manner, she
was tied with strong cords. She was watched for twenty-four
hours, during which time she could not eat or drink. Hopkins's theory was that her imp (small demon) might come in
the shape of a wasp, a moth, a fly, or other insect. Her
observers had to be careful and kill any insect that appeared
in the room. If a fly escaped and they could not kill it, the
woman was judged guilty. The fly was her imp, and she was

sentenced to burn. Hopkins made twenty shillings for each investigation. For example, he made one old woman confess and burn because four flies had appeared in the room, which he considered to be four imps named "Ilemazur," "Pye-wackett," "Peck-in-the-crown," and "Grizel-Greedigut"[14] (figure 12).

For thousands of years, the sinful dangers of bestiality were viewed through the powerful lens of Judaeo-Christianity, and the act was categorized as a form of buggery (sodomy) ("*offensa cujus nominatiocrimen est*"). Animals in bestiality cases were seen as rupturing the divine cosmic order just like animals that harmed humans or were involved in witchcraft (figure 13). Exodus 12:19 declares: "Whosoever lieth with a beast shall surely be put to death," the "whosoever" here referring to both men (Leviticus 20:15) and women (Leviticus 20:16). Other authors have referred to many men convicted of having sexual intercourse with mules, cows, sows, a mare, heifers, and sheep. Goats were the animal of choice for accusations of bestiality combined with witchcraft. Both human and animal were executed, usually by fire but sometimes by beheading or hanging, and their bodies buried together with all legal documents and pieces of evidence.

According to certain rabbinical scholars, the Old Testament Adam had sexual relations with every creature in the Garden of Eden before God created Eve.[15] The most famous tale of animal seduction of a woman is "The King's Daughter

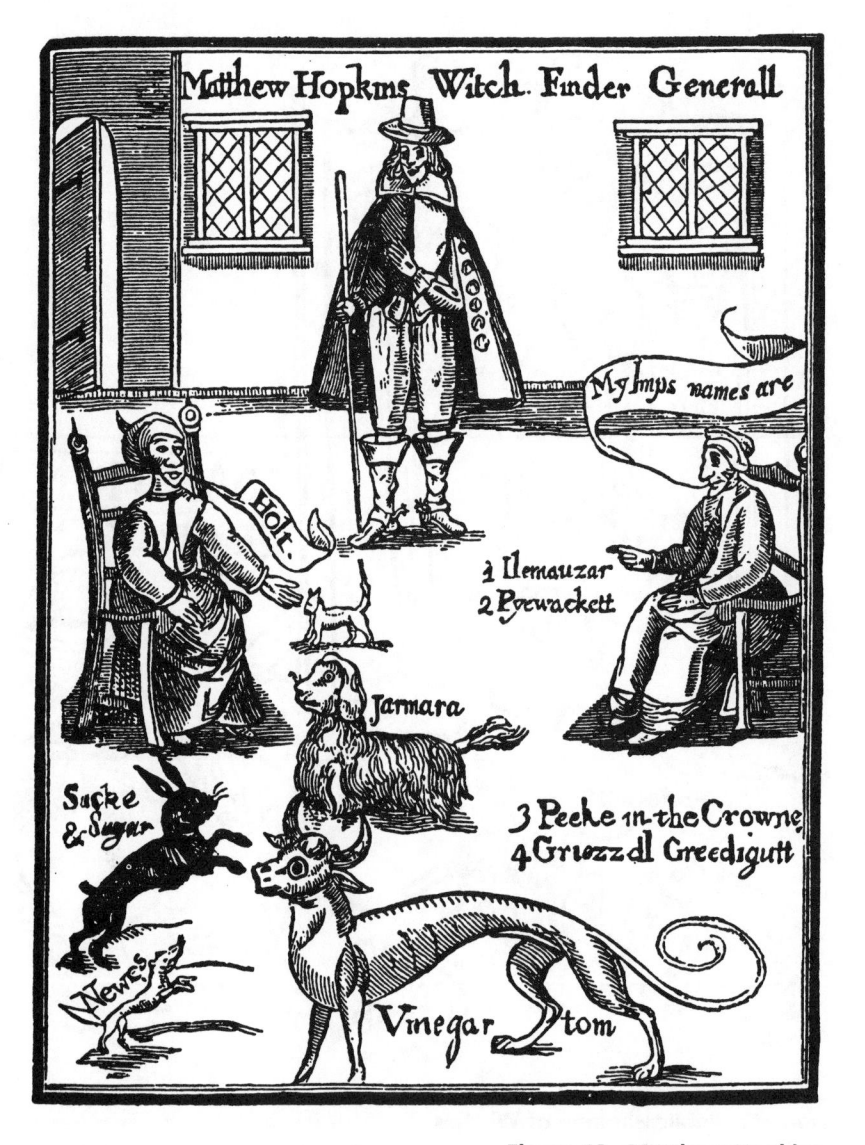

Figure 12. Matthew Hopkins

Searching for a witch's imps is Matthew Hopkins, a seventeenth-century witch-finder. From Charles Mackay, *Extraordinary Popular Delusions and the Madness of Crowds* (New York: Crown, 1995), p. 512.

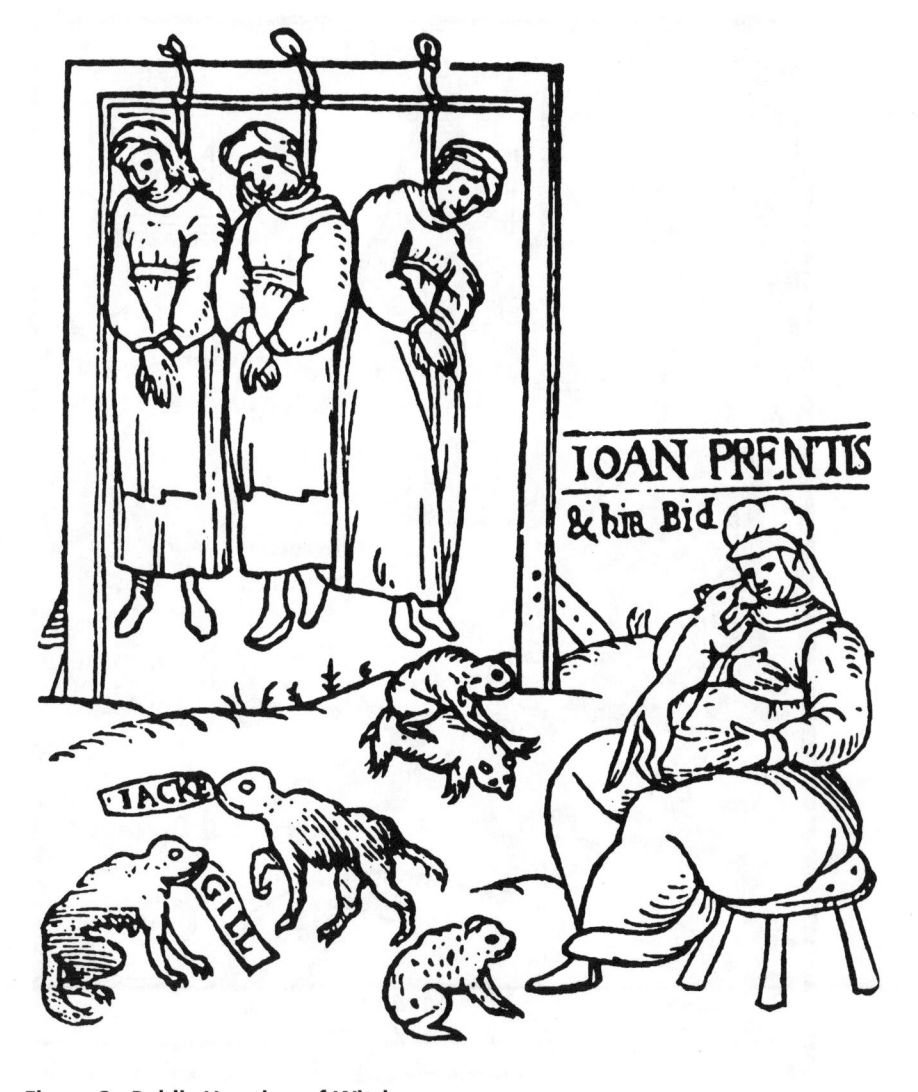

Figure 3. Public Hanging of Witches

The public hanging of three Chelmsford witches, Joan Prentice, Joan Cony, and Joan Upney. From an English pamphlet, 1589. From Ernst Lehner and Johanna Lehner, *Picture Book of Devils, Demons, and Witchcraft*, p. 81, fig. 120.

and the Ape" from the Arabian classic *The Thousand One Arabian Nights*. In his translation, Sir Richard Burton mentions that the ape is probably a baboon, a beast "with a natural penchant for women."

Today many of us abhor bestiality, but some twentieth-century societies have been slow to condemn sexual intercourse with large animals. For example, the Copper Eskimos who used to live on North America's Arctic coast seemed to enjoy intercourse with live or dead animals.[16] Bestiality was also common among the North American Hopi Indians and the Masai of East Africa.[17] Danish explorer Knud Rasmussen recorded the following Eskimo tale:

> There was once a woman who would not have a husband. Her family let dogs copulate with her. They took her out to an island, where the dogs then made her pregnant. After that she gave birth to white men. Before there had been no white men.[18]

After reading the literature on Mary Toft, I wondered why her contemporaries seemed surprised but not *revolted* by the idea of animal sex or animals births. Was bestiality common in England under King George? I doubt it, but the number of societies that have practiced bestiality is mind-boggling, and some may have been known to Mary's contemporaries. Another interesting example were East African fishermen who lived on the coast of the Red Sea and the Indian Ocean. They used to have regular coitus with the carcasses of female dugong (large marine mammals about eight feet in length). The vagina of the dugong is said to anatomically resemble a woman's vagina. The fishermen believed that coitus with the carcass is necessary to "lay the ghost" of the creature; otherwise it might pursue the hunter.[19]

What would it be like to make love to a dead dugong? The idea sends a chill up my spine. The creature usually weighs from 230 to 360 kg (500 to 800 pounds). It has a round, tapered body that ends in a flipper with paired branches. The forelimbs are rounded flippers; there are no hind limbs. The head blends into the body with no visible neck and has a broad, bristled snout. This is not your classic *Playboy* centerfold.

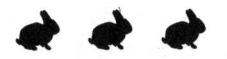

I've often wondered how Mary's vagina could hold such large objects. Do you think she was able to place a rabbit carcass inside herself? The human vagina, when not engaged in intercourse, is often much smaller than a penis. However, the vaginal tissue can obviously expand and can easily double its volumetric capacity when necessary. As author G. L. Simons notes, "It is not always realized, however, how capacious the human vagina can in fact be." In one case reported by

Simons, a woman was encouraged to insert as many coins as possible into her vagina:

> Walter produced five English pounds, all in shillings, and attempted to insert as many coins as possible into the woman's capacious tract. Shilling after shilling he put up her, until forty were embedded in the elastic gully. On and on she went, until no less than seventy coins were inserted. Triumphantly she walked up and down the room, none falling out her vagina.[20, 21]

Even cavemen had sex with animals.[22] One example of Ice Age cave art shows a man on skilike objects while having sex with an elk. Middle Eastern cave paintings suggest that sex with female crocodiles would bring men success in life. The Incas—sixteenth-century South American Indians who ruled a huge empire—had laws preventing llama drivers from having sex with their animals. The Incas enforced these laws by requiring chaperones to escort the llama drivers. The English poet Algernon Charles Swinburne (1837–1909) claimed he had copulated with a monkey. In 1857, Utah soldier Warren Drake was found guilty of having sexual relations with a mare. A court martial sentenced both Drake and the mare to death. The soldier's sentence was commuted to exile from Utah; the less fortunate mare was put to death. I could go on with modern story after story of this type that includes ducks, pigeons, pit bulls, horses, pigs, and raccoons—but you get the point. The idea of Mary having sex with rabbits, or having rabbit children, is not as peculiar as it may sound upon an initial reading.

The educated scientists of Mary's day, of course, had their doubts. Even though respected eighteenth-century scientists did not accept the idea of women birthing animals, there were so many tales in the literature that many learned men were confused. Consider the following examples:

- Dr. John Maubray, a London obstetrician who knew Mary Toft, believed that Dutch women gave birth to molelike animals if the women stayed too close to hot stoves. The creatures were called *sooterkin* (or *sootikin*), and they were described as having short tails and sparkling eyes. While on this odd topic, I cannot help but mention a seemingly related definition of sootikin horrifyingly detailed in Alan Williams' and Maggie Noach's *The Dictionary of Disgusting Facts*. They define a sootikin as a small, mouse-shaped deposit formed in the vaginal cleft of poor women who did not wear undergarments—common until the nineteenth century:

A sootikin built up over several weeks, even months, of not washing. It was composed of particles of soot, dirt, sweat, smegma . . . and vaginal and menstrual discharge. When it reached a certain size and weight, it tended to work loose and drop from under the woman's skirt.

Contemporary writings, including those of English diarist Samuel Pepys (1633–1703) and biographer James Boswell (1740–1795), mention men employed in London churches to sweep up sootikin after services.

- Pliny the Elder (23–79 C.E.) was the Roman savant and author of *Natural History*, an encyclopedic work that was an authority on scientific matters up to the Middle Ages. He wrote of the Roman lady Alcippa who gave birth to an elephant!

- Ole Worm, the famous Danish anatomist, operated a museum in Leyden from 1588 to 1655 that displayed a wide array of biological and anatomical curiosities (figure 14). In his comprehensive *Museum Wormianum*, Mr. Worm described a Norwegian woman who had laid two hen's eggs. One of these fantastic eggs was kept in the king of Denmark's private museum and was finally sold at public auction in 1824.

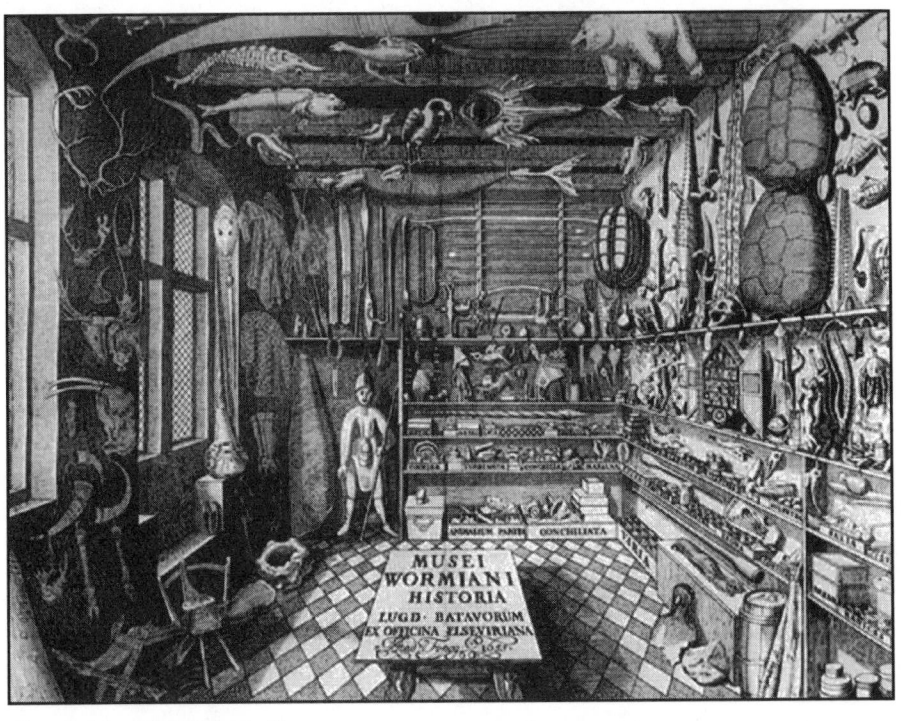

Figure 14. Ole Worm's Museum

People of the 1500s through the 1700s were particularly fond of
biological and anatomical curiosities, as exemplified by Ole Worm's
Museum Wormianum. From Yvette Gayrard-Valy,
Fossils: Evidence of Vanished Worlds (New York: Harry Abrams, 1994), p. 31.

- Thomas Bartholin (1616–1680) was the Danish anatomist and mathematician who was first to fully describe the entire human lymphatic system. He also described a noblewoman from Elsinore, Denmark, who had given birth to a large rat that ran around the room trying to escape once it was ejected from her body.

- In Greek mythology, Pasiphaë, wife of King Minos, fell in love with a snow-white bull and had intercourse with it, and the fruit of this passion was the Minotaur, who had a man's body and a bull's head. Her child by the bull was shut up in the Labyrinth created for Minos by Daedalus. (Incidentally, the ancient Greeks had a number of rather bizarre sexual practices, as described in *Sexual Life in Ancient Greece*.[23])

- St. Peter Damian (1007–1072), church cardinal and doctor, told a famous tale involving animal offspring in his *De bono religiosi status et variorum animatium tropologia*.[24] In this allegedly true story, Count Gulielmus had both a pet ape and a promiscuous wife. In due course, the ape became the wife's lover. One day the ape was jealous when seeing the woman lying with her husband, and the ape attacked the man and killed him. Pope Alexander II showed Damian the offspring of the countess and the ape! The monster, an apelike boy, was called Maimo after his simian father. (Alexander II was pope from 1061 to 1073 and known for his enforcement of clerical celibacy.)

- In 1278, a Swiss woman gave birth to a lion. In 1471, an Italian a woman gave birth to a dog. In 1531, a Spanish woman gave birth to serpents and pigs. The list is endless.[25]

I've just given a number of reasons why people in the 1700s may have been more open to the idea of women giving birth to animals than we are today. There were so many stories circulating on this subject that even wise men may have been predisposed to consider Mary's story plausible. However, a lady had more than one orifice through which she could eject animals. I fondly recall the case of "The Woman Who Vomited Frogs."

In 1642, Mrs. Catharina Geisslerin was widely known as "the toad-vomiting woman of Germany." She told people that she had swallowed tadpoles in swamp water, and that frogs were thriving in her intestinal tract. Whenever she drank milk, the frogs would hop about madly. Despite initial skepticism, she convinced physicians that amphibians were in her digestive system—especially after she vomited fully grown frogs (sometimes living) for two years in front of famous professors and medical consultants!

When Dr. Thomas Rheinesius, a great physician from Saxony, decided to study Catharina's case, she seemed to stop vomiting frogs. He wanted to examine her further, and for three months gave her various foul solutions to encourage her to vomit and have diarrhea. But no frogs came forth. Next, Professor Michaelis from Leipzig came to give Catharina more powerful agents to encourage vomiting—which caused her to vomit a frog leg.

In 1648, after the physicians had left, Catharina began vomiting amphibians with a passion—and the famous Thomas

Bartholin was called in to study her. Bartholin, a student of the Dutch school of anatomists, was no slouch. He taught at the University of Copenhagen (1646–1661) and served as physician to King Christian V.[26] As mentioned previously, Bartholin was the first person to fully describe the entire human lymphatic system. If anyone could solve the mystery of the frog-vomiting woman, he could, or so people thought.

Bartholin started his research by cutting up one of Catharina's frog children. He was shocked to find dozens of black flies inside the stomach. How could this be if the frog had grown to maturity within the woman's belly? Like St. André who did not consider mature rabbit dung and floating lungs indicative of fraud, Bartholin did not think the flies meant Catharina swallowed frogs and vomited them in front of spectators a few minutes later.

When Catharina died in 1662, the medical community was excited about dissecting her body to search for amphibians within her stomach or intestines. To their dismay, the physicians found no creatures. Catharina did not die by amphibian overcrowding but by liver inflammation.

The scientists studying Catharina did not realize that the stomach's digestive juices would quickly destroy amphibians. (The warm temperature also contributes to their demise.)

Throughout the seventeenth and eighteenth centuries, there were many stories of people vomiting amphibians, and most German pathological museums contained vomited amphibians that allegedly lived for years in a person's digestive tract. For example, in 1694, Theodorus Döderlein of southern Germany vomited twenty-one newts and four frogs (figure 15). In 1834, Mrs. Henriette Pfenning vomited frogs in front of applauding crowds of spectators. (She later admitted her hoax—she stashed the frogs inside her skirt pockets and pretended to vomit the frogs.)

Why did these individuals swallow creatures only to vomit (or pretend to vomit) them in front of crowds?[27] No doubt much of it was for attention, although it is possible that obsessive-compulsive disorder played a role in some cases. People afflicted with obsessive-compulsive disorder perform endless odd rituals that dominate their daily lives. For example, trichotillomaniacs continuously pull out their hair. Other people with obsessive-compulsive disorder continually wash their hands, check if a door is locked, perform rituals while going through doorways, and so on. Almost all people afflicted with obsessive-compulsive disorder recognize their problems and therefore often keep their embarrassing diseases hidden.

The most extreme case of compulsive swallowing is that of a forty-two-year-old woman who, in 1927, complained of a "slight abdominal pain." Physicians removed 2,533 objects from her stomach, including 947 bent pins. In 1985, physicians removed 212 objects from a man whose stomach contents included 53 toothbrushes, 2 razors, 2 telescopic aerials, and 150 handles of disposable razors.[28]

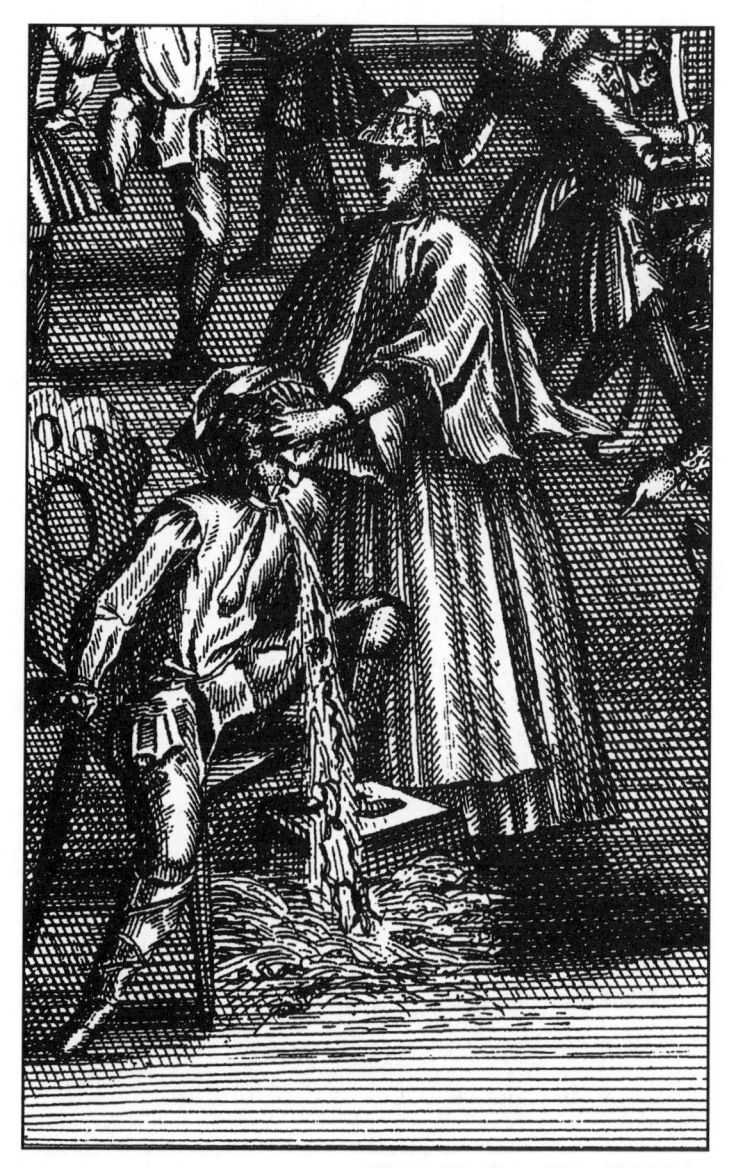

Figure 15. Theodorus Dödelein

From Jan Bondeson, *A Cabinet of Medical Curiosities*, p. 37, fig. 5.
Originally published in Georg Abraham Mercklin, *De Incantamentis*, 1715.

On the flip side of the coin are those individuals who insert objects into their rectums. Modern medical journals list an astonishing array of objects: a bottle of Mrs. Butterworth's syrup, an ax handle, a 9-inch zucchini, a plastic spatula, a Coke bottle, an 11-inch carrot, an antenna rod, a 150-watt light bulb, 72 jeweler's saws, an apple, a frozen pig's tail, an 18-inch umbrella handle, two Vaseline jars, a teacup, an oilcan, a 6-by-5-inch tool box, a two-pound stone, a baby powder can, a peanut butter jar, a ball-point pen, baseballs, a sand-filled bicycle inner tube, sewing needles, a flashlight, a tobacco pouch, a turnip, a pair of eyeglasses, a hard-boiled egg, a carborundum grindstone, a suitcase key, tumblers and glasses, and a polyethylene waste trap from the U-bend of a sink. In 1955, one depressed man inserted a six-inch paper tube into his rectum, dropped in a lighted firecracker, and blew a hole in his anterior rectal wall.[29]

Some strange food cravings are so common today that they have scientific names of their own, for example:[30]

- *pagophagia*—ice eating
- *xylophagia*—wooden toothpick eating
- *coniophagia*—dust eating
- *geophagia*—clay or dirt eating
- *amylophagia*—the consumption of laundry starch and paste
- *coprophagia*—feces eating

Experimental evidence shows that pica, the intentional and compulsive consumption of nonfood substances, can be a sign of iron or other nutrient deficiency, or mental illness. Pica can drive children and adults to exhibit pagophagia, geophagia, and amylophagia, and also the consumption of ash, chalk, antacids, paint chips, plaster, wax, and paint. Pica occurs worldwide and is common among people of either sex and of all ages and races. One sufferer admitted to consuming ice cubes from five ice trays every day, supplemented by bags of crushed ice obtained at convenience stores. Another sufferer followed her husband to collect his cigarette ashes so she could eat them. A significant number of clay-eaters have shown up in emergency rooms with obstructed or even perforated intestines. Many pica sufferers can be cured if they are given iron supplements.

Coprophagia, or eating one's own feces, has been reported in many animals, where it can be either a normal or pathological behavior. Coprophagia in humans is uncommon, and more likely to occur in patients with old age dementia, depression, hypothyroidism, learning disability, and severe psychosis such as associated with schizophrenia in young adults. Coprophagia has been described in many animals including lemur, marmoset, horse, guinea-pig, chinchilla, beaver, and shrew. The growth of rats is stunted by 20 percent when coprophagia is prevented. Coprophagia, a normal behavior in rabbits and rodents, appears to aid bacterial synthesis of nutrients, particularly B group vitamins and vitamin K in the colon.

Feces ingestion is also a feature of a culture-bound syndrome, called Piblokto, in Eskimos (Inuits). In the mentally handicapped, nutritional supplements have reduced the frequency of coprophagia.

Today, our fascination with alien "parasites" continues in the science-fiction literature that describes creatures popping from peoples' orifices. One of the most bizarre examples occurs in Philip Jose Farmer's *Image of the Beast*, in which a snakelike being lives within a woman's vagina and uterus. The creature has the tiny of head of a man:

> A tiny thing, like a slender white tongue, spurted from her slit . . . like a snake or an eel. It kept coming out, and its skin was smooth and hairless. . . . It shot out in a downward arc . . . and then it turned and flopped over against her belly. It continued to slide out from the slit as if yards of it were still coiled inside her womb. . . . Its head was the size of a golf ball . . . with black hair around the tiny ears. . . . The eyes were dark. The woman's lips moved. Childe could not hear, but he thought that she was crooning.[31]

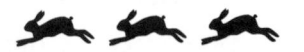

What else could have been going through St. André's mind that would predispose him to believe one animal species might give birth to another? In centuries before, scientists believed an even stranger theory of *spontaneous generation* (or abiogenesis) in which living organisms develop from non-living matter. People observed that cheese wrapped in rags and left in a dark corner spontaneously produced mice. Many believed in spontaneous generation because it explained the appearance of maggots on decaying meat.

By the eighteenth century, it became obvious that non-living material could not produce higher organisms. However, scientists were still uncertain how bacteria arose until Louis Pasteur's nineteenth-century experiments.

The history of the spontaneous generation's downfall is fascinating. In 1668, Italian physician Francesco Redi showed that maggots in putrefying meat did not result from spontaneous generation but from eggs laid on the meat by flies.[32] In one of the first examples of a biological experiment with proper controls, Redi set up a series of flasks containing meats. Half of the flasks were sealed, half open. He then repeated the experiment but, instead of sealing the flasks, covered half of them with gauze so that air could enter. Although the meat in all of the flasks putrefied, Redi found that the meat contained maggots only in the open and uncovered flasks which flies had entered freely. He correctly concluded that the maggots came from eggs laid on the meat by flies. (Despite this evidence, Redi continued to believe that the process of spontaneous generation still applied to intestinal worms.)

The greatest biologist of the nineteenth century was Louis Pasteur (1822–1895), who finally put an end to the idea of spontaneous generation of bacteria. In a simple experiment using a sterilized flask with a bent neck, he showed that pure air cannot initiate the growth of microorganisms. A culture can grow in the flask only if germs enter it. Pasteur concluded that "there is no known circumstance in which it can be confirmed that microscopic beings came into the world without germs, without parents similar to themselves."[33]

Pasteur is remembered for many reasons. He proved that microorganisms cause fermentation and disease. He originated vaccines and was the first to use them for rabies, anthrax, and chicken cholera. He saved the beer, wine, and silk industries of France and other countries. For example, his pasteurization process, which used heat to destroy harmful germs, made it possible to preserve and transport wine and vinegar without their undergoing deterioration. He saved the silkworm industry by isolating the bacilli that infected worms. He performed pioneering work in stereochemistry, and he originated the process known as pasteurization.

It is fascinating to speculate on how medicine's course would be altered had men like Pasteur been transported back in time just one hundred years, say to the time of Mary Toft.

Would he have visited and questioned Mary Toft? How would the state of medicine have been changed *today* as a result of his appearance in 1726? Would people of 1726 have accepted his ideas? Would the British troops have been able to stay healthier and defeat the Americans during the Revolutionary War? What if the French realized Pasteur's military potential and spent one hundred years developing bacterial cultures?[34]

Of course, even tiny changes introduced by Pasteur would have amplified affects through time. This would be true of many minor adjustments in history. As just one example, imagine what would happen if Cleopatra had an ugly but benign skin growth on the tip of her nose. The entire cascade of historical events would be different. A mutation of a single skin cell caused by the random exposure to sunlight could have changed the universe. This entire line of thinking reminds me of a passage from writer Jane Roberts:

> You are so part of the world that your slightest action contributes to its reality. Your breath changes the atmosphere. Your encounters with others alter the fabrics of their lives, and the lives of those who come in contact with them.[35]

NOTES

1. Stephen J. Spignesi, *The Odd Index* (New York: Plume, 1994), p. 205. The *Weekly World News* is available on newsstands everywhere, but if you want to subscribe, write them at P.O. Box 1286, Des Moines, Iowa 50340–1286. Also see their fine web page at: http://weeklyworldnews.com/

2. Joel Achenbach, *Why Things Are and Why Things Aren't* (New York: Ballantine Books, 1996), p. 94.

3. G. L. Simons, *Simons' Book of World Sexual Records* (New York: Bell Publishing Company, 1975), p. 154.

4. Ibid.

5. Ibid., p. 155.

6. A. Edwardes and R. E. L. Masters, *The Cradle of Erotica* (New York: Odyssey Press, 1970), p. 9.

7. Simons, *Simons' Book of World Sexual Records*.

8. Ibid., p. 156.

9. Gaston Dubois-Desaulle, *Bestiality: An Historical, Medical, Legal, and Literary Study*, translated by "A. F. N." (New York: Panurge, 1933).

10. Charles Mackay, *Extraordinary Popular Delusions and the Madness of Crowds* (New York: Farrar, Straus, and Giroux, 1932), 483.

11. Dubois-Desaulle, *Bestiality*, p. 58.

12. Mackay, *Extraordinary Popular Delusions and the Madness of Crowds*, pp. 501–502.

13. Marvin Harris, *Cows, Pigs, Wars, and Witches* (New York: Vintage Books, 1974), p. 211.

14. Mackay, *Extraordinary Popular Delusions and the Madness of Crowds*, p. 512.

15. Simons, *Simons' Book of World Sexual Records*, p. 157.

16. C. S. Ford and F. A. Beach, *Patterns of Sexual Behavoir* (New York: Eyre & Spottiswood, 1952), p. 148.

17. Simons, *Simons' Book of World Sexual Records*, p. 157

18. K. Rasmussen, "Intellectual Culture of the Copper Eskimos," in *Report of the Fifth Thule Expedition*, vol. 9 (Copenhagen: Glydenalske Boghandel, Nordisk Forlag, 1932): pp. 1–350.

19. Simons, *Simons' Book of World Sexual Records*, p. 158

20. Ibid, p. 70.

21. E. and P. Kronhausen, *Walter, the English Casanova* (Polybooks, 1967), p. 238.

22. Karl Shaw, *The Mammoth Book of Tasteless Lists* (New York: Carroll and Graff, 1998), pp. 311–12.

23. H. Licht, *Sexual Life in Ancient Greece* (Abbey Library, 1971), pp. 318–28. As one reviewer noted, "this book will shake your foundation if you thought you knew about ancient Greek sexuality. What some civilizations consider unnatural, others consider wholly natural and beautiful. You may not like what you read, but if you cherish ancient Greek culture, this book gives insight into their sexual practices."

24. Simons, *Simons' Book of World Sexual Records*, p. 156.

25. Dubois-Desaulle, *Bestiality: An Historical, Medical, Legal, and Literary Study*, p. 51.

26. King Christian V (1646–1699) was the Scandinavian king who consolidated "absolutism" in Denmark-Norway. Popular with the common people, he fortified the absolutist system against the aristocracy by accelerating his father's practice of allowing Holstein nobles and Danish commoners into state service. To accommodate them, Christian V created the new noble ranks of count and baron.

27. In my novel *Chaos in Wonderland* I discuss a race of beautiful, translucent, women (called *Reobatrachus*) with strange sexual practices. After the male has fertilized the female's eggs with his sperm, the female swallows the eggs and broods them in her stomach. The nurturing female stops feeding during the breeding period so that the stomach acid does not destroy the eggs. To be more precise, the egg capsules secrete a prostoglandin that stops the mom's stomach from secreting hydrochloric acid. The stomach is transformed from a digestive organ into a protective gestational sac! When it is time for the babies to be born, the mother's esophagus dilates and the young creatures are shot from her mouth. Although readers of *Chaos in Wonderland* found this idea hard to swallow, I had to remind them that the idea of a stomach serving as both a digestive and reproductive organ was inspired by the reproductive strategies of certain frogs on Earth that use their stomachs as reproductive organs. See, for example, W. Duellman, "Reproductive Strategies of Frogs," *Scientific American* (July 1992): 80–87.

28. Donald McFarlan, *The Guiness Book of World Records* (New York: Bantam, 1991), p. 38.

29. For a more comprehensive list of objects people have voluntarily placed inside themselves, see Cecil Adams's *More of The Straight Dope* (New York: Ballantine, 1994).

30. Ibid., p. 91.

31. Philip Jose Farmer, *Image of the Beast* (Chicago: Playboy Press, 1979), p. 117.

32. Redi had read William Harvey's earlier speculations that insects, worms, and frogs do not arise spontaneously, as was then commonly believed, but from seeds or eggs too small to be seen.

33. René Dubos, *Louis Pasteur: Free Lance of Science* (New York: Da Capo Press, Inc., 1959), p. 187.

34. Historian Greg Kishi from Tucson, Arizona, replies:

> What if the French during Mary Toft's age realized Pasteur's military potential and spent one hundred years developing bacterial cultures? What if the French assigned their Foreign Legion to collect tissue samples from dying people in Africa, or if the French used anthrax? World War I starts, and the French use anthrax and cholera instead of mustard gas. Given the dirtiness of the World War I trenches, this would have a devastating effect on the enemy. If the French victor used bacterial warfare, and the German vanquished did not, we would not have the Warsaw Convention guidelines preventing such atrocities today, and the French may have maintained their military advantage. Would the Germans have been able to recover quickly and decimate London, given superior German delivery technology coupled with biological weaponry?

Historian Mike Hocker from Poughkeepsie, New York remarks:

> To imagine the long-range effect of Pasteur's transport to Mary Toft's time, recall that World War I trenches were extremely filthy. A simple razor cut was often fatal (never mind the machine gun bullets, artillery, poison gases, trenchfoot, etc.). Penicillin did not appear until late World War II, and

the Axis was enthusiastic to capture any penicillin stocks. Only recently have military casualty rates from disease been less than combat casualty rates. During World War II the Japanese on the Pacific islands suffered appalling casualties due to disease and starvation, and the American disease casualty rates frequently exceeded casualties due to combat in the island jungles.

If the French used biological warfare early, the Bolshevik revolution would have failed. The major reasons for the revolution were extraordinarily high Russian mortality and morbidity on the front, and starvation of the populace "supporting" the war effort.

The French would inoculate their civilians quickly to prevent collateral damage. Animals might also be susceptible to the disease agents. (Horses were considered war material through World War II; high livestock death rates would lead to human starvation even if all civilians were inoculated. Livestock loss would also slow down the war effort through lack of transport and food since World War I was not very mechanized).

Also keep in mind that biological warfare has been used for millennia. For example, the bodies of plague, smallpox, and typhus victims were lobbed into besieged cities; and smallpox-infected persons and articles were deliberately introduced to Native Americans to decimate the tribal members.

One difficulty of biological weapons is that they sometimes work slowly. Troops that realize they are infected are likely to be very angry and deadly since they have nothing to lose.

35. Jane Roberts, *Seth Speaks* (New York: Amber-Allen, 1994).

CHAPTER FIVE

CHAOS IN THE PUBLIC BATH

I believe that scientific knowledge has fractal properties, that no matter how much we learn, whatever is left, however small it may seem, is just as infinitely complex as the whole was to start with. That, I think, is the secret of the Universe.

—Isaac Asimov, *I. Asimov*

For science, presumably the temple of ultimate truth, fraud can be a deadly intruder; it survives by destroying the great mutual trust that scientists must share.

—The Editors of *Hoaxes and Deceptions*

I never did give anybody hell. I just told the truth and they thought it was hell.

—Harry S. Truman

AT FOUR O'CLOCK IN THE MORNING ON NOVEMBER 28, 1726, Sir Richard Manningham heard an insistent knock on his door. Manningham—Fellow of the Royal Society and one of the greatest living obstetricians—had a feeling who it might be. Outside his London home it was pitch black. When Manningham opened the door, he heard the plaintive cry of an owl as brisk winds whipped the leaves into a frenzy.

On the doorstep were St. André and Mr. Limborch, a German surgeon, dressed in heavy coats.

"Sir," St. André said, "you have received my message?"

"I did."

"Then I beg you to come with us to Guildford to study Mary Toft. King George says we must do it at once. You are to examine her and then we are to bring her back to London."

Manningham nodded and grabbed his coat.

St. André, Manningham, and Mr. Limborch arrived in Guildford at noon that day. Manningham seemed to have an impartial attitude as he carefully investigated the case. Here is what he concluded after examining Mary:

- Her breasts gave a small quantity of "thin serous matter like milk."
- Her stomach was soft and showed no signs of pregnancy.
- Her vagina contained nothing unusual.
- Her os uteri (the opening between the uterus and vagina) was closed tightly.
- Her right side exhibited a slight hardness around her fallopian tube. Perhaps the uterus contained something.[1]

Manningham placed his hand on Mary's belly. "I'd like to feel her abdominal movements. I've heard much about them."

Unfortunately for Manningham, Mary's belly was still.

Howard stepped closer. "Perhaps the rabbit baby inside her has died."

"Perhaps."

Howard reached for some clothes. "Sir Mannigham, sometimes we have been able to cause abdominal contractions by applying hot cloths to her body."

Mannigham nodded. "Do so."

When Howard and St. André applied hot cloths to Mary's belly, her contractions and pulsations started immediately. The motions were strong, especially on the right sight of her body. But she delivered no baby.

Manningham and St. André went to the local White Hart Inn for a break. In less than an hour, Howard came to them waving a crumpled paper containing a horrible-looking organ. A few drops of liquid fell upon the oak table at which Manningham and St. André sat.

"Look!" Howard said, "I took this from Mary. It's the placenta of her latest rabbit child. This is more evidence of Mary's miracles."

Manningham was not one to withhold his opinions. "You should have called *me* for the delivery," he said. "In any case, it looks more like half a hog's bladder than a placenta." Manningham looked closer at the strange membrane. "Smell it. It stinks of urine."

Howard looked down. "No, this is part of the chorion, and I have more at home."

That night, Manningham examined Mary and found the membranes inside her and the opening to her uterus still tightly closed. Again he pulled out something that resembled a hog's bladder.

Manningham turned to Howard and St. André. "This membrane never came out of the *uterus*. Now, get me a hog's bladder to compare this to."[2]

John Howard was able to quickly find a hog's bladder. (Isn't it odd that he happened to have a hog's bladder on hand?) The bladder so closely resembled Mary's membrane that Manningham grew very suspicious. "I will not be convinced about these births' authenticity until I take a membrane out of the *uterus* itself."

St. André and Howard pleaded with Manningham to be more patient, and Mary began to cry, perhaps because Manningham did not believe the births were authentic.

Manningham turned to St. André and Howard, "Tell me, does it not *look* like a hog's bladder. Does it not *smell* like a hog's bladder?"

St. André and Howard hesitantly admitted that the hog's bladder resembled Mary's mystery placenta. Both had the same urinous smell that typified a hog's bladder. (I tried to verify that a hog's bladder smelled like urine, but unfortunately none of the butchers I contacted had a hog's bladder.)

Their conversation was interrupted by Mary, who screamed on and off for three hours but delivered nothing.

Later that day, St. André, Howard, and Manningham returned to the White Hart Inn where their discussions became heated. Because St. André thought Mary could give birth to rabbits, it was not an imaginative stretch to consider she could gave birth to a hog's bladder. He believed that Mary's rabbits and were sufficiently different from normal rabbits that they had to come from her body. "Mary's rabbits are monstrous," St. André said. "They did not come from the woods by her home."

"I am not convinced," Manningham replied.

Worried about damage to his reputation, St. André asked Manningham to withhold any reports until further study. Manningham agreed to the delay because he was confused about Mary's abdominal pulsations and had a haunting suspicion there was something in her uterus. He also thought it possible that Mary had managed to place something (e.g., rabbit parts) into her uterus. In any case, the great Manningham did not delay because he was concerned about St. André's reputation.

On November 29, 1726, the authorities confined Mary to a public bath in Leicester Fields so they could study her more carefully and in a controlled setting. The bathhouse was centrally located in England and not far from St. André's apartments at Northumberland Court. St. André and others hoped that Mary would soon deliver her eighteenth rabbit.

St. André wrote a late-night letter to James Douglas, a highly respected anatomist, famous surgeon, and specialist in the anatomy of women's pelvic organs. In his letter, St. André implored Douglas to come quickly and study Mary. When Douglas arrived at the bathhouse, he found himself with many eminent men, including Claudius Amyand, Sergeant-Surgeon in Ordinary to George I, as well as Manningham, Howard, and St. André.

At this point in the Mary Toft mystery, the public revered St. André and Howard for taking charge of the situation. The public was also in awe of Mary Toft. Perhaps they were also a little bit frightened. After all, she was the young lady who did something no other woman could—she was a prolific rabbit breeder.

In contrast to St. André and Howard, James Douglas was a more methodical man who believed the rabbit births to be a hoax. He argued that neither experience nor science supported the assertion that a human could give birth to animals. Since the uterine structure prevented a woman from shoving rabbits into it from the vagina, he believed that Mary secretly placed them into her vagina when the spectators were not looking.

While at the bathhouse, James Douglas felt Mary's abdominal pulsations. He turned to St. André. "These do not appear to be the motions a woman exhibits when in labor. They're just contractions of the abdominal muscles."

"But—"

"We shouldn't discuss the matter further until a rabbit is born without without the chance of anyone secretly giving her one in the bathhouse."

What started as a scientific study soon degenerated into a circus. Noblemen from around the country came to visit Mary at the bathhouse. Some were motivated by scientific curiosity. Others were lechers who wanted to examine her private parts. Mary tried to satisfy everyone's needs, although she was not happy that she had been brought to London.

Lord John Hervey, the great British politician, wrote:

> Every creature in town both men and women have
> been by to see and feel her. All the eminent physi-
> cians, surgeons, and men-midwifes in London are
> there day and night to watch her next production.[3]

Newspapers provided daily updates on Mary's condition for those who could not visit the bathhouse.

Can you imagine what happened to people who made their living raising and selling rabbits for human consumption? Prices plummeted and many rabbiters went out of business. The public horror was so great that the rent of rabbit warrens (enclosures) virtually ceased. People not only stopped eating rabbits because they had lost their taste after hearing about Mary, but there was also an old law *prohibiting* eating anything that came from a woman during birth, including placenta, umbilical cords, and now—rabbits.

Let us digress a moment and discuss placenta eating. This strange law against placenta eating was enacted during the time of Queen Elizabeth I, who was queen of England from 1558 to 1603. I have not been able to determine why such a law was enacted during a time when Elizabeth's blend of shrewdness, courage, and majestic self-display inspired loyalty and helped unify England against foreign enemies. Historians justly call the latter half of England's sixteenth century "the Elizabethan era," but, alas, they do not mention the strange law forbidding human placenta eating—although a placenta does not appear to be so appetizing that many would flock to it!

Today human placenta stew is enjoyed by the strong of stomach, and I'm told that the stew smells like liver.[4] In her 1978 blockbuster book *Hygieia: A Woman's Herbal*, Jeannine Parvati[5] describes the joys of placenta cuisine:

> It was after a very powerful birthing. The mother ate some raw first; and then let me take some into the kitchen for fixing. My experience of this slab of meat was amazing. I had never felt such life-force present in meat before. . . . This meat still felt very much alive to me as I began to slice it and sauté it in garlic and oil. . . . By the time the placenta was tender, the birthday party members were very hungry, and exhausted. After the supper, eaten in a glowing silence, everyone was energized, very much revitalized. . . . Notwithstanding, the first time I ate placenta has also been my last time. . . . Guess I just lost the taste.
>
> When you first encounter the meat, remember to pause—placenta can be sacred food if you let the meat tell you how to prepare it for the fire. . . . Chew slowly, till the placenta becomes a liquid ambrosia. Placenta is a rare privilege for most of us.

The placenta-eaters rationalize their consumption by telling us placentas contain valuable nutrients. (I do not know if scientific tests bear this out, but it would seem easier to just take a vitamin.) Cat and dog moms eat their placentas, and a chemical in the placentas may stimulate uterine contractions. Jeannine Parvati suggests that American Indians had a variety of placenta rituals, although none of the tribes apparently went so far as to eat placentas.

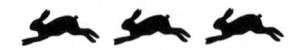

Returning to Mary Toft's tale, we find that during November and December 1726, plays and "obstetrical farces" included scenes in which harlequins, dressed as women, gave birth to pigs and sooterkin. These harlequins made the audiences laugh and reminded them of Mary Toft. In short, England was going wild over Mary's story.

But all was not debauchery at Mary's public bath. Great scientists, physicians, and midwives joined St. André and Howard to study Mary. Dr. John Maubray, the London obstetrician who believed in the sooterkin creatures, also came along to study Mary. He was ecstatic because Mary's babies supported his theory that nonhuman sooterkins could be born from women.

As we discussed, some physicians of the era suggested that a pregnant woman's emotions and longings could transform her embryo into an animal. They thought that Mary's strong desire to eat rabbit meat was a possible cause of her strange children. Dr. Maubray even suggested to pregnant women that they must not play with "dogs, squirrels, and apes" because they risked their children being born resembling these creatures.[6] He also remarked, "If a mouse, rat, weasel, or cat leaps suddenly upon a woman that has conceived, or if an apple, pear, or cherry fall upon any part of her body, the mark of the thing is instantly imprinted [on the fetus]." Midwifery texts dating to the late 1660s clearly spell out the odd effects of emotions on the developing fetus:

> When a mother beholds one with six fingers, she brings forth the like. Or when she sees any thing cut up or divided with a cleaver, she brings forth a divided part or harelip.

During Mary's time, some physicians thought that a mother touching her tongue to a plum could cause the baby to have a plumblike deformity on its tongue. Women who contemplated Jesus's crucifixion too often or intently could produce children with marks on the hands or with other symbols of crucifixion. Watching the slaughter of livestock could give rise to disemboweled children. Playing with rabbits could give rise to children with the long hairy ears. On the other hand, if a mother was surrounded by beautiful things, the child would be beautiful. It's scary to think how much blame these theories placed on the mother for the developmental and physical problems of her infant.

Even the book of Genesis emphasized the idea that visual events in the mother's life affected the offspring's genetics, and some of Mary's physicians were familiar with the story of Jacob. In chapter 30 of Genesis, Jacob devises a scheme to increase his wealth while working for his father-in-law, Laban. The two reached an agreement whereby Laban would give Jacob all striped, spotted, and speckled lambs and kids subsequently born in Laban's flocks. Laban then removed all the striped, spotted, and speckled animals from his flocks and put them in his sons' care at a three-day distance from the flock Jacob attended. Not to be outsmarted, Jacob devised a plan:

> Then Jacob took fresh rods of poplar and almond and plane, and peeled white streaks in them, exposing the white of the rods. He set the rods that he had peeled in front of the flocks in the troughs, that is, the watering places, where the flocks came to drink. And since they bred when they came to drink, the flocks bred in front of the rods, and so the flocks produced young that were striped, speckled, and spotted.

The editors of *The New American Bible* added this interesting footnote to this passage:

> Jacob's stratagem was based on the widespread notion among simple people that visual stimuli can have prenatal effects on the offspring of breeding

animals. Thus, the rods on which Jacob had whittled stripes or bands or chevron marks were thought to cause the female goats that looked at them to bear kids with lighter-colored marks on their dark hair, while the gray ewes were thought to bear lambs with dark marks on them simply by visual cross-breeding with the dark goats.

We know today that animal coloration is a matter of genetics, but the authors of Genesis did not know about genetics, so to them the story made good sense.

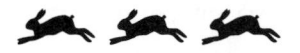

As much as Dr. Maubray accepted the rabbit births as authentic, Manningham and Douglas were skeptical. They decided that Mary must be kept under constant surveillance—all night, all day—to ensure that there was no way she could get rabbits from the outside and fake their births. Of course, these two great physicians couldn't stand watch all by themselves, so they enlisted the help of the local nobility.

Can you imagine how Mary must have felt? She was a poor, uneducated woman under constant surveillance by famous men. On one hand she was probably amazed and even happy for some of the attention. On the other hand, it was a living hell to be constantly watched like an animal in a zoo,[8] even while using the toilet or bathing.

When in the bathhouse, Mary's labor pains came no more. Manningham passed around the hog's bladder she had given birth to, and it became a revered item. It was touched and handled so much that it became worn out, like an old football used for dozens of games.

Because Mary had no more babies, Manningham and Douglas believed they had proof of a scam and decided to announce their opinions to the world. However, St. André and Howard put a stop to their announcement. "Wait," St. André said. "Please give her a little more time. Another miracle will surely take place soon."

St. André started to prevent learned men from studying Mary in favor of leering men who were more accepting of his theories than were Manningham or Douglas.

Sadly, by now Mary Toft was badly infected and had convulsions that few thought were faked. Once she even had a seizure that made her lose consciousness for over two hours. For several days she was cared for and observed by Howard, St. André, Manningham, and often by Douglas.

On Thursday, December 1, Mary seemed to be seized by pains. Manningham examined her and asked Douglas to check her out. Douglas reached in to her vagina and found nothing. Manningham believed the labor pains to be authentic, that something was in her uterus. Douglas thought the labor was faked.

Again St. André and Howard did their best to shape

public opinion by excluding skeptics from the bathhouse. Thomas Brathwait, a famous surgeon, was let in to see Mary on December 1 but when he disagreed with St. André and Howard regarding rabbit anatomy, they didn't let him back in to see Mary.

Chaos in the bathhouse reached a fever pitch when St. André showed Douglas a rough draft of his A Short Narrative of an Extraordinary Delivery of Rabbits. Douglas was not impressed, calling it "nothing but a collection of impossiblities." He told St. André that there was no way rabbits could develop to maturity in the fallopian tubes as St. André argued. Douglas also scoffed at St. André's speculation that the noises he heard were rabbit bones snapping in the womb.

Other investigations were underway behind the scenes. Lord Thomas Onslow, a famous justice of the peace, went to Guildford to investigate some of the local rabbit sellers. Onslow determined that Joshua Toft often purchased young rabbits during his wife's "pregnancies." Joshua claimed they were for Mary to eat, but Mrs. Mason, the owner of the house where Mary stayed, stated she never once cooked a rabbit for Mary Toft while she cared for Mary.

Onslow also learned that Joshua had previously come across some very small rabbits for sale. Joshua had approached a seller in the market. "I'd like to buy these rabbits," Joshua said.

The owner of the rabbits turned to Joshua. "But these are too small for eating."

Joshua shook his head, "I must have them, even if they are small."

In another incident, a rabbiter's rabbit had died the night before and had been thrown out in the trash. Joshua had wanted it anyway: "If you had not thrown it away, it would have done as well for me as a live one."

Onslow also discovered that Joshua frequently talked to his sister Margaret Toft about Mary, and Onslow felt that Margaret acted as a conduit for the rabbits from Joshua to Mary Toft.

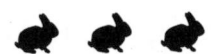

On the cold morning of December 4, a vague perpetual cloud floated in the sky as Mary started having violent labor pains. A hush fell over the bathhouse spectators. Manningham, Maubray, and German obstetrician Dr. Limborsch all seemed to believe that something would come out of Mary any minute. St. André and Howard beamed and strutted with delight. They would at last be vindicated.

"Wait," whispered Thomas Howard, a porter at the bath-house. "She gave me money to get a rabbit for her!" Unfortunately for Mary Toft, Thomas Howard would soon tell Sir Thomas Clarges, justice of the peace, that Mary *bribed* him to bring her the smallest rabbit he could find.[9]

Manningham and Douglas kept the porter's information

quiet, saving it for later, perhaps to suddenly spring on Mary and force a confession. They also wanted hard evidence of a hoax and felt that the porter's information alone would not sufficiently convince the public and kill any interest in Mary Toft's outlandish story. In short, Manningham and Douglas were looking for the "smoking gun," not just circumstantial evidence.

Meanwhile, there was a new, chilling development that made Manningham especially confused. While Mary was still in labor with violent contractions, Manningham was shocked to see a swelling above her "os pubis."

"Something will soon come from the uterus!" Manningham shouted.

What in God's name could it be? Mary had been carefully watched to eliminate all possibility of fraud. At no time was she alone. Even the great Douglas was surprised by the swelling and could not explain it.[10] St. André and Howard were jubilant with the latest development and confidentially told the crowds gathered in the bathhouse that something would soon be born.

Alas, all signs of labor soon went away. Mary soon became quiet and limp, like a wilting flower.

On the evening of December 4, Sir Thomas Clarges, Justice of the Peace, was called to the bathhouse. Thomas Howard, the porter, swore that Mary bribed him to purchase a small rabbit.

Clarges took Mary Toft into custody and began a harsh interrogation. The sequence of events follows:

- Mary denied everything, and Clarges dismissed her.
- Clarges called in Mary's sister-in-law Margaret who admitted that Mary had asked the porter to get a rabbit.
- Clarges questioned Mary Toft again, and she insisted she had only wanted to *eat* the rabbit.
- Clarges decided to throw Mary into prison for deceiving the public and creating a national hysteria.[11]

"Please," Manningham said to Clarges. "Let Mary stay at the bathhouse a little longer so I can obtain irrefutable evidence of the hoax. If you put Mary in prison, the story will be kept alive in the public's mind." Manningham wanted to continually watch Mary in the bathhouse and worried that in jail she could not be observed by the various surgeons.

From that moment on, Mary was continuously attacked from all sides and pressured to confess. Today, any confession given under such dire conditions would be meaningless in the same way that coerced confessions under torture are meaningless. Nevertheless, Clarges threatened her, Manningham and Douglas repeatedly coaxed her to tell the truth, and The Duke of Montagu and Lord Baltimore told her to confess.

Mary maintained her story that the rabbits procured for

her were to cook and eat. "I truly am pregnant with rabbits right now," she said.

Manningham waited another two days but was now thoroughly impatient. He began his harshest interrogation of Mary yet. To me it seems cruel that he threatened to send chimney sweeps to look into her uterus and fallopian tubes. "Mary," Manningham said. "We will perform very painful operations and experiments on you to discover your secret."[12]

With sobs in her voice, Mary asked to think about Manningham's threats. If she did not confess by the next morning, she would allow Manningham to slice her open and study her private parts.

On the morning of December 7, Mary was taken before Sir Richard Manningham, James Douglas, Lord Baltimore, and the Duke of Montague. "I will not go on any longer thus," she said. "I shall sooner hang myself."

Her confession was taken down and is preserved to this day among James Douglas's files at the Hunterian Library in Glasgow. However, her first rounds of confession did not sound plausible. Mary said that soon after her August miscarriage she met a strange woman who suggested the entire scheme of giving birth to rabbits.

The next day, Manningham and Douglas put pressure on her to be *entirely* truthful, and Mary gave up the story of the mysterious stranger. This time she said her mother-in-law Ann Toft was responsible for the hoax. Mary asserted her own innocence and thought she had actually given birth to rabbits! She also hinted that Mr. Howard worked with Ann Toft.

Some authors[13] suggest that Mary also confessed she had hidden dismembered rabbit carcasses in a specially-designed pocket located in her skirt. Whenever she was not closely watched, she introduced them into her vagina. In the beginning, she was amazed that she could deceive such famous men as St. André. After she had placed the rabbit guts into her vagina, she would go into a false labor, move her abdomen, yell, and finally give birth to the pieces.

We will never know the entire truth because no confession given under such conditions can be totally credible. But what Mary said was sufficient for her to be charged with being a "Notorious and Vile Cheat," and on December 9 she was thrown into Bridewell, a prison for beggars and tramps. She would spend her Christmas behind bars looking out at evergreens coated with a patina of snow that glimmered like mercury. Occasionally strangers, young and old, would point up at her window, people whom Mary could never know.

If Mary Toft lived today, I doubt she would be thrown in prison. What crime did she actually commit that would land her in jail? In our modern world where TV shows like *The X-Files* are among the most popular, in which characters routinely see visions of the Virgin Mary in office building windows, listen with rapt attention to gurus who channel spirits, or see statues weep, what would happen if a woman today claimed to give birth to rabbits? Would she be immediately dismissed as a nut or charlatan? Or would she be hailed as the next guru of enlightenment?

Let us assume that Mary Toft concealed rabbit parts in her clothes and placed them in her vagina while no one looked. If you think such a deception could not possibly take place in our modern world, consider the "psychic surgeons" who hide chicken guts in false thumbs and then appear to perform bloody operations, removing "tumors" from peoples' abdomens. As discussed in James Randi's book *Flim Flam*,[14] sleight-of-hand artists in the Philippines, Brazil, and now all over the world use simple deceptions to give the impression that they are actually placing their hands within the human body, without making incisions, to remove tumors. These hoaxers are not only able to convince the gullible public, but also several physicians, just like in St. André's time!

When filmed, these psychic surgeries usually start with an obese person lying on his back. An incision seems to appear when the psychic surgeon runs his finger along the abdomen. A stream of blood spurts from beneath the surgeon's hands.

Pieces of guts appear and are tossed away. Finally, the surgeon mops up the blood with some cotton wadding, and no incision remains.

When scientists brought blood samples back to their labs, they found the blood to be from a cow. The "tumor" is a piece of chicken intestine. When the psychic surgeons are confronted, they claim that the miracle is even greater because the human tumors are transformed into animal tissue! Echoes of Mary Toft abound.

James Randi's remarks about today's psychic surgery have startling relevance to the Mary Toft case:

> How is it all done? Certainly there is lots of blood, and chicken guts don't just come from nowhere, do they? No, no more than the magician's rabbit comes from nowhere. I recall the remark of one magician who was asked how he pulled a rabbit from a hat. "Well," he said, "the first thing is to get the rabbit *into* the hat."[15]

The first thing that the psychic surgeon does is purchase a false thumb available at many magic-trick shops. The thumb is filled with blood and chicken intestines before the operation. During the operation, the thumb is pulled off to permit blood to flow, along with bits of chicken intestines. The fake thumb is then returned to fit over the real thumb. Finally the false thumb is picked up in the cotton wadding and discarded.

When performing, the psychic surgeons appear to reach inside the body with their fingers penetrating the stomach. This is easily accomplished with fat people when the surgeons' fingers are curled up and the knuckles pressed into the skin. Try this yourself on your spouse or friend. It gives a distinct impression that the fingers are passing through the skin. Note, however, that when a psychic surgeon himself needs surgery, for example for an appendix removal, he goes to traditional surgeons in hospitals.

Despite the evidence, there are still noncritical believers of psychic surgery. European medical practitioner Sigrun Seutemann suggests that Philippine faith healers can perform *genuine* surgery with their bare hands. She notes that one of them, Tony Agpaoa, usually placed wet cotton wool on the body, and red liquid comes out of the cotton. The operation lasted three to seven minutes. She writes:

> This type of operation seems to be an astral materialization. Examination of the specimens that have been removed and of the blood shows them to be human or animal. . . . Tony's fingers disappear inside the body. He does not open the body with his fingertips, but with the first joint of his fingers—this could give the impression that he was hiding something in his hands. I have investigated all possibilities of fraud and could find none. . . . I have never seen any trickery. . . . I think these phenomena cannot be explained in terms of the science of today. Even examination of the blood and tissue specimens removed does not relate to the results of

normal surgery because the protein seems to change as a result of the healer's vibrations. Healing occurs in cases which have not responded to normal methods; healing also occurs with some hopeless cases. This in itself is proof that the healers are not using faked techniques.[16]

Brazil's Jose Arigo (1921–1971) was another famous psychic surgeon. Known as the "surgeon of the rusty knife," he claimed to perform surgery with little pain, blood, or infection. Despite tales of his skill, subsequent research showed that Arigo only performed primitive surgeries like lancing boils or removing cysts while prescribing antibiotics.[17]

If we in the 1990s can believe in psychic surgery that does not obey physical laws, it is not too much of an imaginative stretch to understand how medical men of the 1700s could believe in women giving birth to rabbits.

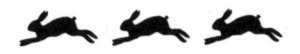

Back to Mary's story. St. André had published his *Short Narrative* on December 3, the same day the bathhouse porter revealed Mary's bribe to bring her a rabbit. Perhaps St. André thought that his publication would discredit the porter's story. Whatever his motive, it seemed to be a last-ditch effort to make the whole affair seem more believable. St. André promised to write another paper that carefully compared Mary's babies to normal rabbits. Alas, this was never to happen. On December 8, he published a retraction in which he admitted his belief that Mary had perpetrated a hoax:

> Having contributed, in some measure, to the belief of an impostor, in a Narrative lately published by me of an extraordinary delivery of rabbits, performed by Mr. Howard, Surgeon of Guildford; and having been since instrumental in discovering the same; so that I am now thoroughly convinced it is a most abominable fraud: I think myself obliged, in strict regard to the truth, to acquaint the public thereof; and that I intend, in a short time, to publish a full Account of this Discovery, with some considerations on the extraordinary circumstances of this case, which misled me in my apprehensions thereof; and which as I hope they will, in some measure, excuse the mistakes made by myself, and others, who have visited the woman concerned therein, will also be acceptable to the world, in separating the innocent from those who have been guilty actors of this fraud.[18]

St. André never wrote his full "Account of this Discovery."

Sir Richard Manningham worried that the public blamed *him* for initially withholding his opinions, so on December 12, he published *An Exact Diary of What Was Observed During a Close Attendance Upon Mary*. He gave all the details of the deception, as far as he understood them, and emphasized his role in discovering how Mary accomplished her miraculous births.

Contrary to what the various physicians hoped for, they brought more suspicion on themselves by rushing to publish all their notes, letters, and pamphlets of self-vindication. The goal of all the scientific players was to publish papers to make them appear *less* foolish in the eyes of King George and the public. For example, Cyriacus Ahlers, the German surgeon on staff to King George, feared that St. André's *Short Narrative* would severely damage his reputation. Therefore, Ahlers published his own pamphlet *Some Observations Concerning the Woman of Godlyman* emphasizing the gullibility on John Howard. Ahlers wrote that Howard had examined Mary while in a nightgown and while assuming "indecent postures"—with salacious implications. Ahlers went so far as to suggest that Howard was in collusion with Mary Toft. After all, both Ahlers and St. André offered Howard money.

Cyriacus Ahlers felt a special need to exonerate himself after St. André called him a hypocrite and told everyone Ahlers promised Mary a pension from the king. Ahlers explained that he had suspected a hoax from the beginning, especially after examining the rabbit dung consisting of corn and other vegetation.

Other physicians wrote concerned letters that the Toft scandal damaged the reputation of all British physicians. One popular work, *The Anatomist Dissected* by "Lemuel Gulliver," personally attacked St. André and other involved doctors for their gullibility. There were other publications, attributed to Jonathan Swift (1667–1745) (the author of *Gulliver's Travels* published in the same year), that were alleged to be Mary's true confessions.

Thomas Brathwait, the famous surgeon who saw Mary once in the bathhouse but was subsequently turned away, published *Remarks on a Short Narrative of and Extraordinary Delivery of Rabbits*. By all accounts, it was a well-reasoned analysis. The public ate it up—in fact they were attracted to all the publications like flies to dung. It was as big a story as Marilyn Monroe's or Watergate. Within a week, Brathwait's *Remarks* went into a second edition. *The Anatomist Dissected* went into a third printing. St. André's much earlier pamphlet describing an assassination attempt on his life was reprinted. People circulated flyers that contained the full text of Mary Toft's alleged suicide note. The forgery said she had cut her throat from ear to ear. Many people in London were angry with Mary, and satires depicted her with an uncontrollable yearning for the penis. In one such satire, "Mary Toft" writes in her own words: "I wos a Wuman as had grate natturul parts and a large cpassiti."

Even John Howard, whose behavior seemed exemplary,

was satirized, and he promised to publish "a particular account of all that occurred to my knowledge, relating to Mary Toft of Godalmin." The account was never published.

Mary Toft continued to portray herself as an innocent victim. Mary claimed she was intimidated into perpetrating the scam by her ruthless mother-in-law, Ann Toft, who helped engineer the idea. Mary further suggested that her husband was completely uninvolved with the hoax and should not be persecuted. Most likely Mary and her husband were closely involved from the beginning, because it would have been impossible to pull it off without collaborating. (Recall that Joshua had purchased many baby rabbits.) Margaret, Joshua's older sister, also probably played a role in passing rabbits from Joshua to Mary.

Dennis Todd, author of *Imagining Monsters*, suggests Mary got the idea for the hoax after she actually gave birth to a deformed fetus in the summer of 1726.[19] In her confession, she said that she miscarried a large, misshapen piece of flesh, and for about a month afterward suffered from occasional heavy bleeding. This may have given Mary the idea of giving birth not to rabbits, but to a monster she confessed to creating by cutting up a cat and inserting into its intestines the backbone of an eel she had eaten for dinner. She had shoved the unwholesome mess into her vagina, and then sent for the neighbor Mary Gill.

Mary also said that early in the scam, Ann Toft had put a

rabbit's jaw and skull into her, causing great pain and bleeding. The Tofts had not planned for the hoax to focus on rabbits, but with the delivery of the rabbit skull, they felt committed. They were no longer delivering monsters but rabbits.

Recall St. André's initial "proof" of Mary's genuineness when she delivered a fur ball and rabbit head while he watched her closely, keeping his hand in her vagina to eliminate fraud. (If you don't recall, reread chapter 3.) How could Mary have tricked him? In her confession, Mary said she had hidden both the fur and the head in her vagina before St. André came into the room. Mary said that St. André made "a very slight examination" of her. Perhaps in his haste, or in his desire to believe or for fame, he had carelessly overlooked the obvious. After all, this was to be his ticket to European stardom.

Just like today's O. J. Simpson case or the media coverage of President Clinton's sex scandal, the press during the time of Mary Toft went wild. Londoners talked of little else during the winter of 1726. They scarcely followed more important news of state affairs.

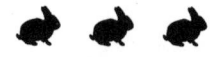

I wonder what effect the Mary Toft story would have had if it had taken place six years earlier during the South Sea Company scandal. The South Sea Company, which was founded in 1711 to trade (mainly in slaves) with Spanish America, suffered a financial collapse in 1720. In the ensuing scandal it became apparent that King George and his mistresses had taken part in South Sea Company transactions of questionable legality, but George's strong-willed ministers skillfully handled the House of Commons and saved the king from disgrace. As a result, King George was forced to give his ministers a free hand in the ministry. They pushed several of the king's friends out of office, and by 1724 the king had come to rely completely on their judgment.

The public interest in Mary Toft was so great that there was renewed interest in female anatomy, and words like "uterus" and "fallopian tubes" were commonly known even to the uneducated. In 1726, Writer William Stratford described interest in the story:

> The rabbit affair is as great a monster in its kind as any, even this age, has produced. . . . It has given an occasion to the ladies of our age to show their modesty, in talking modestly upon it such things as their mothers would have thought an affront to them to have had any spoke in their presence.[20]

As we already discussed, there was an explosion of coverage of the Mary Toft case in pamphlets, papers, and even ballads. (Today we would get similar coverage in our tabloids and news magazines.) Most of these stories made St. André appear to be an idiot. Others continued to make fun of Mary's sexual organs. Famous British poet and satirist Alexander Pope (1688–1744) even published a bawdy song that was popular in the alehouses. John Laguerre exploited public interest by publishing a mezzotint[21] depicting Mary Toft seated in a chair and holding a rabbit in her lap (see figure 4, p. 38).

The Scottish mathematician, physician, and writer Dr. John Arbuthnot (1667–1735) satirized Lord Peterborough, a well-known lecher, by implying Peterborough was the rabbits' father:

> The Doctor searched both high and low,
> And found no rabbit there.
> But peering nearer cried, Soho,
> I'm sure I have found a hare.
>
> They all affirm with one accord,
> When they had searched her thorough,
> That bunny's dad must be a lord,
> Whose name does end in burrough.

By the 1800s, the many pamphlets and poems about Mary had become quite valuable to collectors. Complete collections bound in rabbit skin were sold for fifteen to twenty guineas. (A guinea is a gold coin issued in England from 1663 to 1813 and worth one pound and one shilling.) Today the

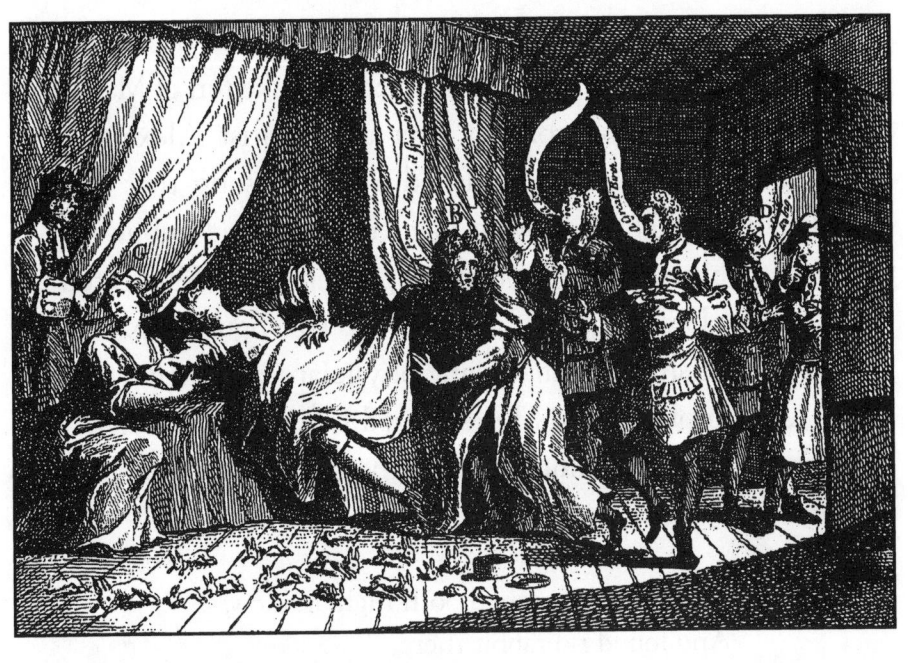

Figure 16. *Cunicularii, or The Wise Men of Godliman in Consultation*

Depicted from left or right are the amazed Joshua Toft, Mary's sister-in-law Margaret Toft, Mary Toft herself, Sir Richard Manningham (wearing a large black wig) searching in Mary's vagina, Dr. Maubray screaming "A Sooterkin!" and St. André dancing with a violin. At the door, John Howard tells a rabbit seller to go away, saying, "It's too big!" By William Hogarth, 1726.

various artifacts command extravagant prices at rare book auctions. Several collections of pamphlets, poems, articles, and letters are kept at the Bodleian Library in Oxford, the Waller Library in Upsala, and the Library of the Royal Society of Medicine in London.

A few months after Mary's hoax was discovered, several

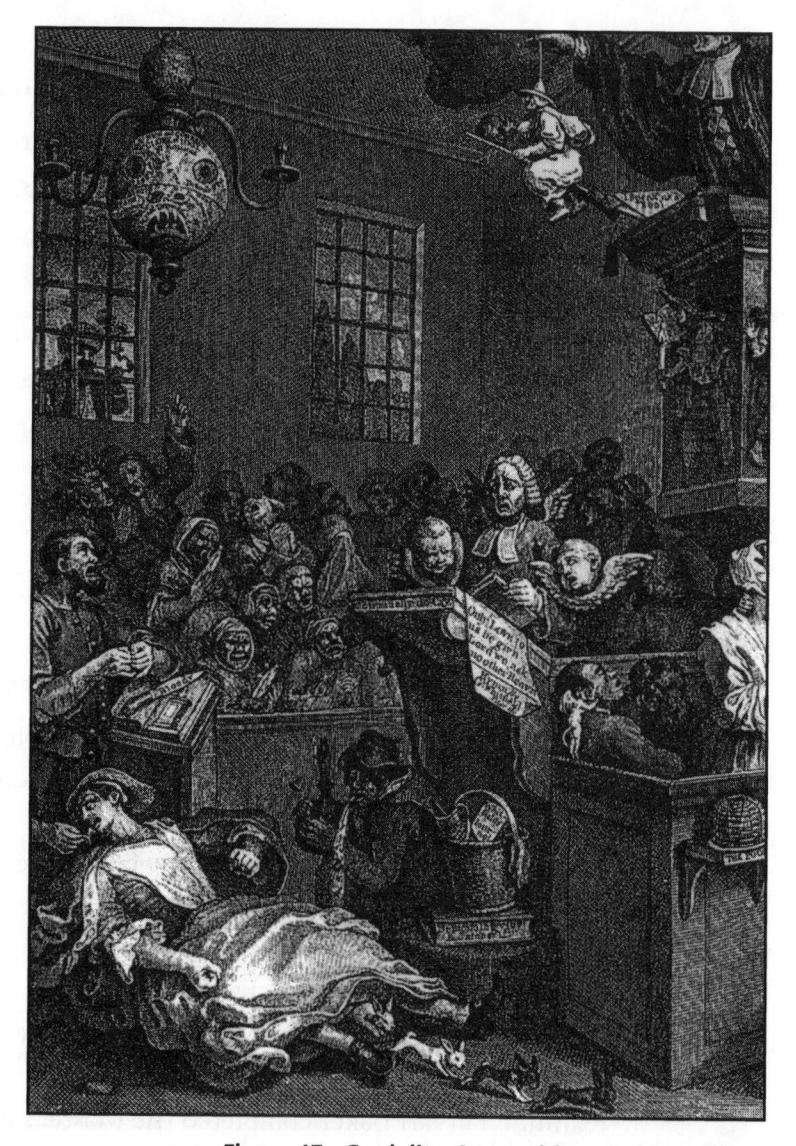

Figure 17. *Credulity, Superstition, and Fanaticism*

Mary is on the floor giving birth to rabbits hopping beneath her dress.
Next to her is the nail-vomiting Boy of Bilston, who perpetrated a hoax
in which he made people believe he was bewitched. By William Hogarth, 1762.

London doctors decided that a caricature should be made to commemorate the Mary Toft affair. Everyone at the dinner contributed one guinea to the cause, and an engraving was made from a zany sketch by William Hogarth (1697–1764), the first great English-born artist to attract admiration abroad.[22] (See figures 16 and 17.)

Hogarth believed that British people had a history of being far too gullible and caught up in some deception. To Hogarth, Mary Toft's tale was an allegory of national unease and of self-delusion.

NOTES

1. Sir Richard Manningham, "An Exact Diary of What Was Observed During a Close Attendance upon Mary Toft, the Pretended Rabbet-Breeder of Goldaming in Surrey" (London, 1726), pp. 10–11.

2. Some authors like Jan Bondeson seem to place the hog-bladder scene at a London public bath, while others, such as Dennis Todd, have it taking place in Guildford.

3. Lord Hervey to Henry Fox, December 3, 1776.

4. Cecil Adams, *Return of the Straight Dope* (New York: Ballantine, 1994), p. 105.

5. Jeannine Parvati Baker completed the Master's program in psychology at Sonoma State University and is the founder of Hygieia College, devoted to "healing the Earth by healing birth." She is the author of *Prenatal Yoga and Natural Birth*, *Hygieia: A*

Woman's Herbal, and *Conscious Conception.* Jeannine is in private practice in central Utah.

6. John Maubray, *Female Physician* (London, 1724), pp. 62–63.

7. Peter Cole, *Culpepper's Directory for Midwives* (London, 1662), p. 146.

8. Mary was uncomfortable under constant surveillance, but her problems were nothing compared to a more disturbing nineteenth-century medical saga. In the summer of 1822, a French Canadian named Alexis St. Martin suffered a gunshot wound to his stomach. Dr. William Beaumont, a young army surgeon stationed at Michigan's Fort Mackinac, rushed to the scene. In his journal he wrote:

> In this dilemma I considered any attempt to save his life entirely useless. But as I had ever considered it a duty to use every means in my power to preserve life when called to administer relief, I proceeded to cleanse the wound and give it superficial dressing, not believing it possible for him to survive twenty minutes.

Without modern antibiotics or anesthetics, Dr. Beaumont was able to nurse St. Martin back to health. However, St. Martin's wound healed with a permanent hole, or fistula, between the stomach's interior and the abdominal wall. Dr. Beaumont persuaded him to become a living laboratory, his belly serving as a cutaway model of the stomach's anatomy and functioning. While watching St. Martin's stomach at work, Beaumont produced very accurate and useful descriptions of stomach functions. Unfortunately, St. Martin, who was sufficiently healthy to work and raise a family, didn't want to be a guinea pig. He craved an independent life free of constant medical observation. *Smithsonian* magazine reviewer Donald Dale Jackson writes:

> The demanding, self-righteous physician and the unlearned, irresponsible patient came to loathe each other. Despite a contract that obliged him to "obey, suffer and comply with all reasonable or proper orders or experiments" in return for room, board and cash, St. Martin fled, only to be coaxed back and then to flee again. When he died, twenty-eight years after Beaumont's death, his financially strapped family was determined to leave him in peace at last. They turned down doctors' requests to autopsy the body and exhibit the celebrated stomach.

Today Dr. Beaumont is generally recognized as the father of American physiology. Alexis St. Martin, the subject of his research, lived to age eighty-three. For more information on similar medical cases, see James Thomas Flexner's *Doctors on Horseback* (Fordham University Press, 1993). For insightful commentary on *Doctors on Horseback*, see Donald Dale Jackson's review in *Smithsonian* 25, no. 10 (January 1995): 122–25.

9. In some accounts, Thomas Howard, the porter, did not volunteer the information about being bribed to bring Mary a rabbit until *after* he was caught. Also, in some accounts this alleged bribery came to light slightly before December 4.

10. The next day Howard attributed Mary's swelling to "flatulent humours."

11. Dennis Todd, *Imagining Monsters* (Chicago: Chicago University Press, 1995), pp. 32–33.

12. Ibid., p. 32; Jan Bondeson, *A Cabinet of Medical Curiosities* (Ithaca, N.Y.: Cornell University Press, 1997), p. 133.

13. Bondeson, *A Cabinet of Medical Curiosities*.

14. James Randi, *Flim-Flam* (Amherst, N.Y.: Prometheus Books, 1981).

15. Ibid., p. 180.

16. Dennis Milner and Edward Smart, *The Loom of Creation* (New York: Harper & Row, 1976), pp. 249–50.

17. Joe Nickell and Matt Nisbet, "Miraculous Surgery," *Skeptical Inquirer* 22, no. 6 (November/December 1998): 15.

18. St. André, "Retraction," *The Daily Journal* (December 9, 1726).

19. Dennis Todd, *Imagining Monsters*, p. 6.

20. William Stratford to Edward Hasby, December 20, 1726, *Historical Manuscripts Commission: Report on the Manuscripts of His Grace the Duke of Portland, K.G.* (London: Machie & Co., 1901); Todd, *Imagining Monsters*, p. 281.

21. A mezzotint is a method of engraving a metal plate by pricking its entire surface with numerous holes that will hold ink and, when printed, produce large areas of tone. The term mezzotint, from Italian mezza tinta or "halftone," derives from the capability of the process to produce soft, subtle gradations of tone.

22. Hogarth is best known for his moral and satirical engravings and paintings such as *A Rake's Progress* (eight scenes, begun

1732). His attempts to build a reputation as a history painter and portraitist, however, met with financial disappointment, and his aesthetic theories had more influence in Romantic literature than in painting.

CHAPTER SIX

WHATEVER BECAME OF MARY TOFT?

It's silly to go on pretending that under the skin we are all brothers. The truth is more likely that under the skin we are all cannibals, assassins, traitors, liars, hypocrites, poltroons.

—Henry Miller (1891–1980)

And whatsoever goeth upon his paws, among all manner of beasts that go on all four, those are unclean unto you: whoso toucheth their carcase shall be unclean until the even.

—Leviticus 11: 27

Age cannot wither her, nor custom stale
Her infinite variety; other women cloy
The appetites they feed; but she makes hungry
Where most she satisfies.
—William Shakespeare, *Anthony and Cleopatra*

MARY TOFT WAS THE MONICA LEWINSKY OF THE 1700s. Both women elicited an avalanche of media coverage, jokes, and national shame. Monica's story cast a bad light on American politics; Mary's affair placed the eighteenth-century London physicians in a bad light. Many of the doctors were ignorant and self-serving—caring only about their reputations and fame, and how to best win favor with the king and royalty. With today's Internet, Mary's story would spread across the world in minutes and would be believed by those whose mental immune systems have not been strengthened by exposure to medical hoaxes. There would be newsgroups like alt.fan.mary-toft and web pages offering the very latest gossip.

Although today few have heard of Mary Toft, interest occurs in isolated media pockets from time to time. For example, in a 1997 issue of the *New Yorker* there is fleeting reference:

In November of 1726, an Englishwoman named Mary Toft became briefly famous when she claimed she had given birth to rabbits. . . . Mrs. Toft was regarded with particular interest in contemporary scientific circles. If true, her tale would prove that (as some had suspected) a woman with a sufficiently vivid imagination could be impregnated by the force of her own desires. She was investigated by several leading medical men of the day. Cyriacus Ahlers, one of the royal surgeons, assisted her in the delivery of yet another rabbit, a stillbirth, and took its skin away to show to King George I. On December 7, Mrs. Toft confessed to having faked the births, and on December 11 an enterprising young man named William Hogarth published a satirical print lampooning all those involved, which he entitled "The Cunicularii, or the Wise Men of Godliman in Consultation."[1]

Professor Howard M. Solomon from Tuft University's History Department discussed the Mary Toft mystery in his fall 2000 class titled "Deception and Identity in Early Modern Europe." Here is a description of the fascinating course:

History 181-HWW, Deception and Identity in Early Modern Europe

If historians cannot be absolutely sure of the motives of saints and heroes, then how do we make sense of out-and-out frauds, liars, and cheats? This seminar will wrestle with that dilemma, exploring the role of fraud and deception in early modern Europe, 1550–1789. We will examine a number of case studies from French and English sources, in order to come to some conclusions about the institutional role of fraud and deception in social, political, and cultural life. These include: politics and statecraft (the construction of the Sun King myth during the reign of Louis XIV; John Law's "Mississippi Bubble" scheme; Monsieur d'Eon, a transvestite diplomat in the court of Louis XV; Marie Antoinette and the Diamond Necklace Affair); personal identity and peasant culture (Arnauld du Tihl, the fraudulent husband of a sixteenth century peasant woman; Mary Toft, an illiterate woman from Surrey who announced in 1726 that she had given birth to seventeen rabbits); rumor and fantasy (rumors of disappearing children in Louis XV's Paris; carnival and masquerade as opportunities for social protest); medicine and science (witches, monsters, and the "scientific revolution").

Scholars still wonder how Mary Toft got the idea of giving birth to rabbits. We discussed the possibility that her (alleged) summer miscarriage gave her the idea, but no one knows for sure. It may be that she had heard about Dr. Maubray's theory of sooterkins, the little dark beasts. It's even possible that John Howard read about sooterkins and helped Mary plan the hoax. At the time, many people thought Howard was a co-conspirator, but Howard was possibly just a scapegoat. Mary may have gotten the idea from tales of women giving birth to animals—tales which persist to this day in the tabloid newspapers and on TV shows like the *X-Files*. During her confession, Mary claimed that the hoax was motivated solely for money so that she could escape her terrible poverty. Mary had confessed she did it "to get so good a living that I should never want as long as I lived."

We already know that on December 9, 1726, Mary was put in jail for her role in the hoax. To prevent any more rabbit births, Joshua Toft was carefully searched whenever he visited. However, Mary's imprisonment did little to dampen public fascinating. The *London Journal* wrote, "Infinite crowds of people . . . resort to see her." For six months, no one talked about anything else.

The case against Mary was eventually dismissed. Perhaps the authorities thought her time spent in Bridewell was sufficient punishment for deceiving the nation. Perhaps they thought that releasing her would help the story die and repair reputations.

Again, we can ask ourselves one of this book's central questions: Why did so many people believe her? Mary Toft's story was compelling because it touched on our basic beliefs and fears—our anxieties about having deformed children, of being deceived, of losing control, of being helpless pawns in the hands of uncaring scientists, of revealing the chilling gullibility of "great" men in whom we place trust. Many educated people who believed her story because eminent men, like St. André, said it was possible. Many who visited Mary in the bathhouse went away true believers. Many members of the parliament believed Mary Toft.

Even priests and other religious figures became mired in the scandal. William Whiston (1667–1752), the famous Anglican priest who sought to harmonize religion and science, told Molyneux that the rabbit births fulfilled Esdras's prophesy foretelling the Final Judgment. (The Second Book of Esdras,[2] written around 100 C.E., describes a future age and humankind's final disposition.) Whiston's remarks made Molyneux quite nervous. Several decades after Mary confessed to the hoax, William Whiston was still arguing that she really had given birth to rabbits.

There were many other men of distinction who were confused by the Mary Toft affair. The Scottish mathematician, physician, and writer Dr. John Arbuthnot (1667–1735) came to see Mary Toft at the bathhouse and initially believed her, although he soon had suspicions and later satirized the affair. In any case, people like Molyneux and Arbuthnot reveal their uncertainty about Mary Toft in various conversations they had with their contemporaries.

Most of the learned men wanted to withhold their final judgment until a long scientific study took place. Even the skeptical James Douglas seemed to consider the *possibility* that Mary Toft could give birth to rabbits:

> You are too well aquainted with the caution that is necessary in examining extraordinary phenomena of nature either real or pretended, and with regard to the reputation of all persons who have the least shadow of any to lose, not to be convinced that my conduct was ever way suitable both to the dictates of philosophy and the obligations of society.... Those laws which nature observes in the formation of the foetus in particular are as yet but very imperfectly known, and it must certainly be a very great presumption in any man from the small insight has into them, to venture to binde the effects thereof any farther than experience directs him.... Recollect the instances of monstrous births already recorded....[3]

Mary's story capitalized on the age-old English fascination with monsters and freaks and their willingness to pay good money to see them. Consider all the dragons and strange "unbiological creatures" that had surrounded people for centuries. For example, there were wild creatures in Ulysses Aldrovandus's *Serpentum et Draconium Historiae* (History of Serpents and Dragons), in which he blurs the line between fact and fiction. Aldrovandus (1522–1605) was a celebrated naturalist of the sixteenth century. His thirteen-volume work on natural history contained a confusing mix of fables and oddities along with valuable scientific information. His book on monsters displayed all the curiosities and monstrosities one could find in nature. In Bologna, he housed one of the richest collections of natural specimens and curiosities in Europe. Figures 18 through 20 show a variety of odd creatures from the fifteenth and sixteenth centuries, many of which depict animal-animal and human-animal hybrids.

Although these kinds of books and illustrations might seem too dated to influence scientists in Mary's time, the images still pervaded the popular culture. Aldrovandus's work went through thirty editions in English and French. Fortunius Licetus's 1634 book *De Monstres* (On Monsters) contained numerous images of malformed animals and humans. He argued that malformations arose from superfetation (fertilization of an egg ovulated during a pregnancy so that fetuses of different ages exist simultaneously in the pregnant female). Ambroise Paré's *Des Monstres et Prodigies* (On Monsters and Prodigies, ca. 1570) presented numerous examples of monstrous births, many of them even wilder than Mary Toft's. Some cases include women bearing frogs, snakes, and eels:

> Monsieur the Count Charles de Mansfeld recently being sick at the hotel de Guise with a high and constant fever, ejected a certain matter similar to an

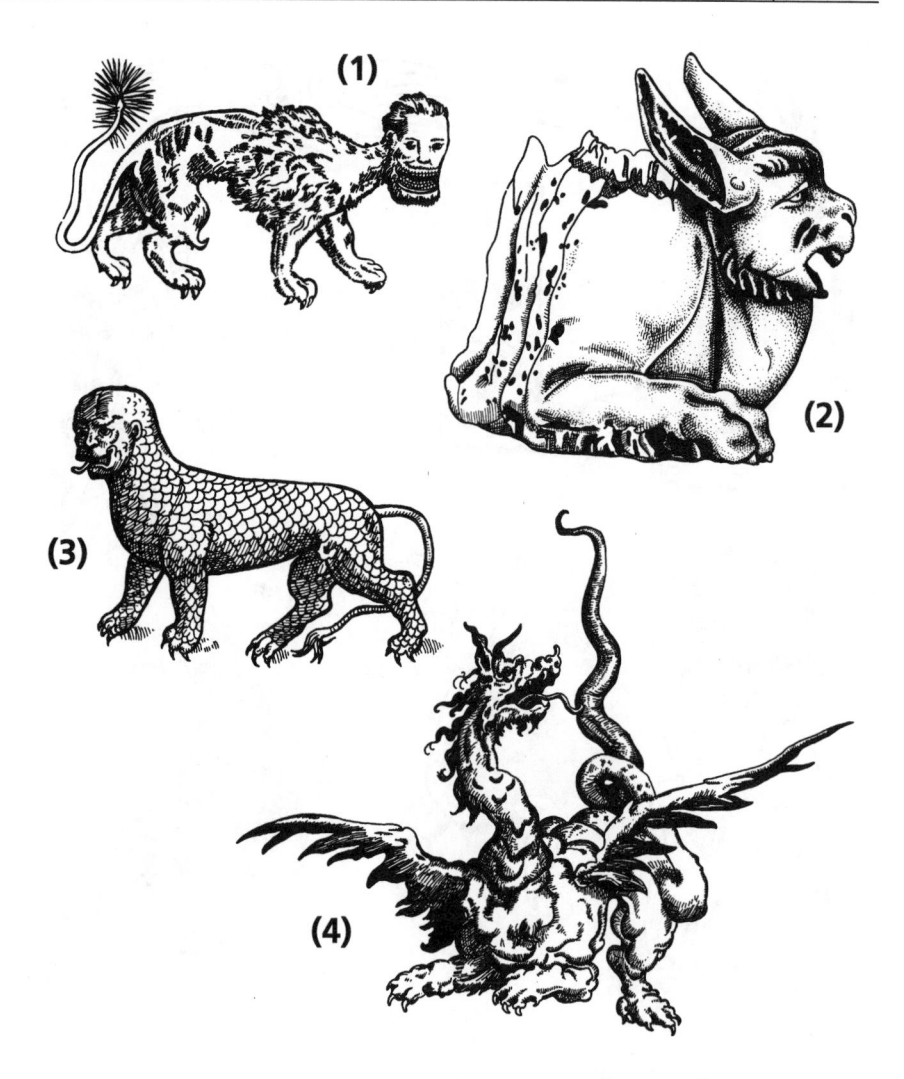

Figure 18. European Beasts, Sixteenth and Seventeenth Centuries

(1) Manitcore, from a woodcut by E. Topsell, 1607. (2) Monster, from a French ivory sculpture, fourteenth or fifteenth century. (3) Lion-fish, from a woodcut, ca. seventeenth century. (4) Dragon, from a French engraving, 1589. From Richard Huber, *Treasury of Fantastic and Mythological Creatures* (New York: Dover, 1981), plate 45.

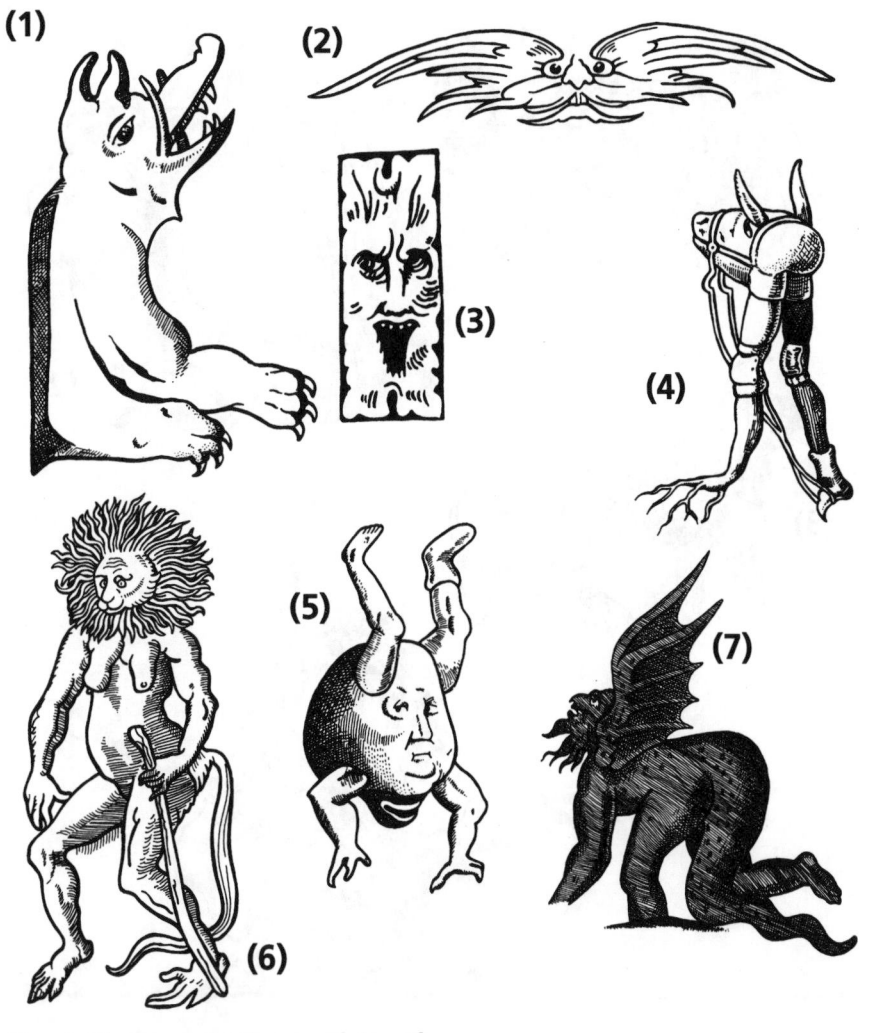

Figure 19. European Beasts, Sixteenth, Seventeenth, and Eighteenth Centuries

(1) Witch's familiar, from a medieval drawing. (2) Winged mask, from an etching by Jacques Callot, 1617. (3) Border design. (4) and (5) Monsters from *The Sabbat*, engraving after Pieter Brueghel the Elder, 1565. (6) Creature from a fifteenth-century woodcut. (7) Satan, from an engraving, probably eighteenth century. From Richard Huber, *Treasury of Fantastic and Mythological Creatures*, plate 51.

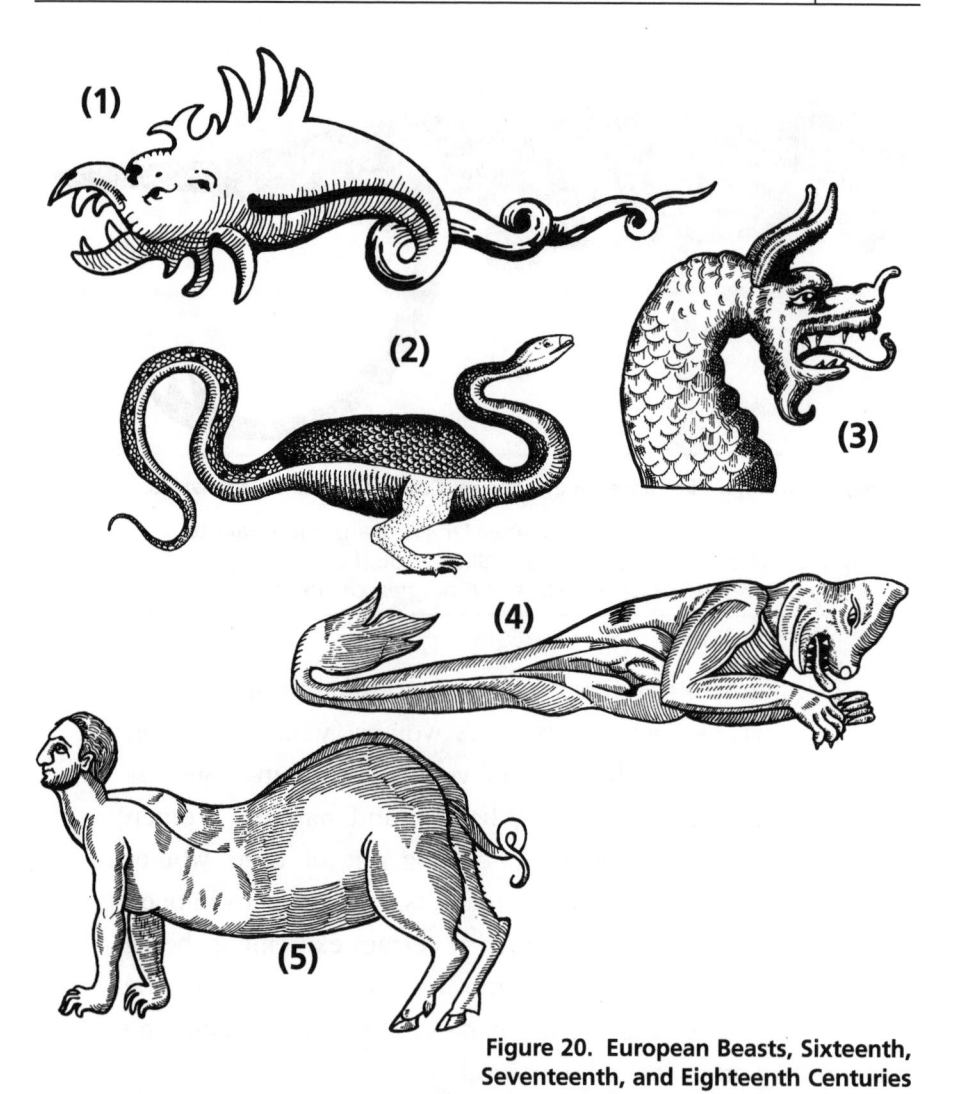

Figure 20. European Beasts, Sixteenth, Seventeenth, and Eighteenth Centuries

(1) Flying demon, from *Abomination of Sorcerers*, by Jasper Isaac, sixteenth century. (2) Lizard-serpent, from an engraving, probably eighteenth century. (3) Dragon's head, from an eighteenth-century print. (4) Sea monster, from a sixteenth- or seventeenth-century woodcut. (5) Pig man from a sixteenth- or seventeenth-century woodcut. From Richard Huber, *Treasury of Fantastic and Mythological Creatures*, plate 62.

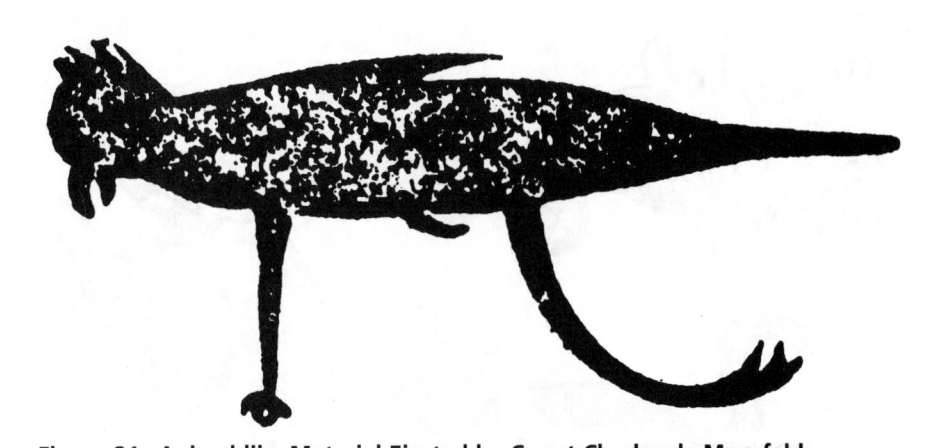

Figure 21. Animal-like Material Ejected by Count Charles de Mansfeld

From Ambroise Paré, *On Monsters and Marvels*, trans. Janis Pallister
(Chicago: University of Chicago Press, 1983), p. 56, fig. 34.
Originally published as *Des Monstres et Prodigies*, ca. 1570.

animal [see figure 21]. Many animal forms are likewise created in women's wombs (which are often found with fetuses and well-formed young), such as frogs, toads, snakes, lizards, and harpies. Women have been observed casting out of their wombs snakes and other creatures, which can happen through the corruption of certain excrements being retained in their womb, as one sees occur in the intestines and other parts of our bodies, thick long worms, indeed hairy and horned.

Paré believed that birth defects arose from God's wrath, too little or too much semen, sodomy, atheism, the mother's bad posture, or the wild imagination of the mother. Paré writes:

There was a girl as furry as a bear, whom the mother had bred thus deformed and hideous, for having looked too intensely at the image of Saint John the Baptist dressed in skins, along with his own body hair and beard, which picture was attached to the foot of her bed while she was conceiving.

Hippocrates saved a princess accused of adultery, because she had given birth to a child as black as a Moor, her husband and she both having white skin; which woman was absolved upon Hippocrates' persuasion that it was caused by the portrait of a Moor, similar to the child, which was customarily attached to her bed.

Moreover, one can observe that rabbits and peacocks who are closed up in white places, through the properties of their imagination, give birth to their white young.

Paré also wrote about a boy with the face of a frog (figure 22). The disfigurement was supposedly caused by the mother who held a frog in her hand while having sex with her husband. I can hear you asking, why was she holding a frog in her hand while enjoying the pleasures of conjugal bliss? The answer is simple. She had a fever, and the neighbors advised her that she could cure her fever by holding a live frog in her hand until the frog died. That night her husband requested sex, but because she still had a fever, she went to bed with her husband and held the frog during

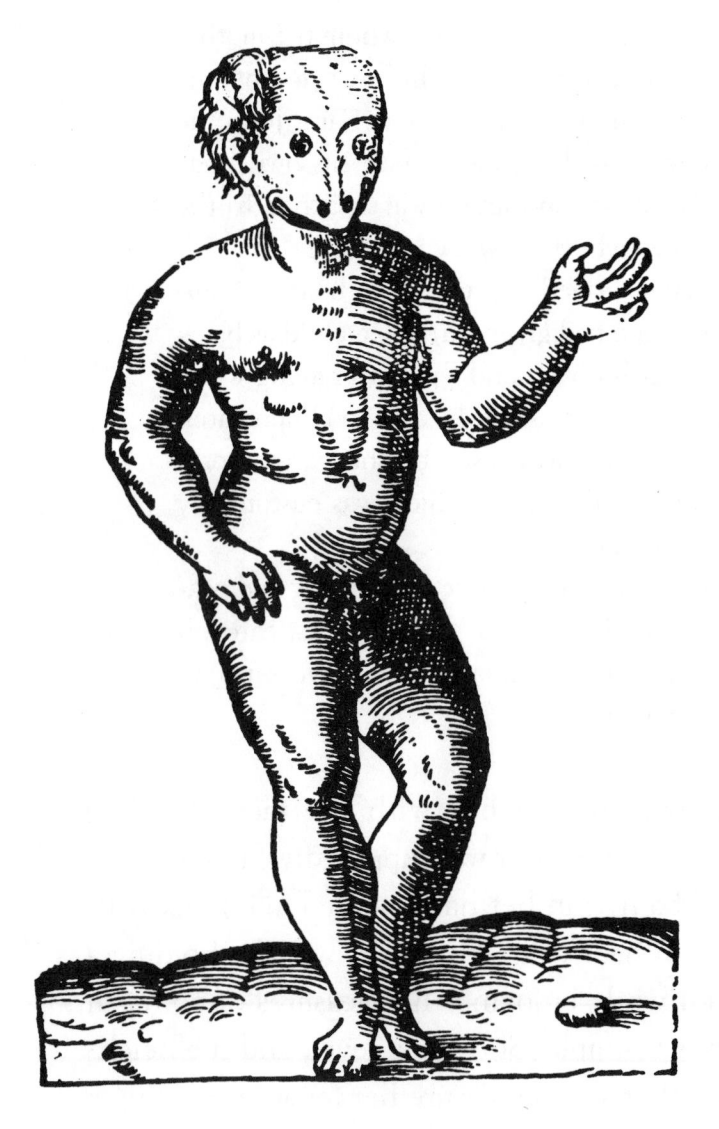

Figure 22. A Child with the Face of a Frog

This child was born with the face of a frog because his mother held a frog while having intercourse with her husband. From Ambroise Paré, *On Monsters and Marvels*, p. 41, fig. 28. Originally published as *Des Monstres et Prodigies*, ca. 1570.

intercourse. I do not know if the husband realized what was in her hand.

Born in France around 1510, Paré eventually became chief surgeon to both Charles IX and Henri III. Surgeons of Paré's time were considered inferior to physicians because surgeons were less educated and made a living using their hands. Physicians often criticized Paré for daring to write about topics beyond his area of specialization. Although Paré made many astute observations, he also passed along many unsubstantiated accounts of sea devils, marine sows, and "monstrous" animals with human faces.

There was an endless number of supposedly authentic "monsters" still available to stimulate people's imagination during Mary's time. Here are a few favorites:

- In 1570, Abraham Ortelius published *Theatrum Orbis Terrarum*. His maps of Iceland show sea monsters with piglike faces that many believed inhabited the surrounding waters.
- In 1572, J. Sluperius drew cyclopses. His sixteenth-century engravings kept alive a myth that started thousands of years before, when ancient Greeks assumed elephant skulls belonged to giants, and the median nasal openings comprised a single eye socket.
- In 1573–1585, Ambroise Paré published *Des Monstres* which contained images of creatures called sea eagles

(figure 23). In actuality, these were "Jenny Hanivers," forgeries made by mutilating a ray to resemble a winged sea monster with a human head. The trick worked, and Ambroise Paré recounted a secondhand tale of how a live specimen was presented to the lords of the city of Quioze (modern-day Chioggia, a town in northern Italy). The origin of the name "Jenny Haniver" is unknown, but the first known illustration of the forged animal dates from the sixteenth century. Paré wrote:

A flying fish was caught that was frightening and gave marvel to see, being four feet and more in length and twice as much in width from one tip to the other of its wings, and a good square in thickness. Its head was wondrously thick, having two eyes, one on top of the other, in a line; two large ears and two mouths; its snout was very fleshy, green in color, its wings were double; on its throat it had five holes; its tail was long, on top of which were two little wings. It was brought quite alive to the city of Quioze, and presented to the lords of this later, as a thing that had never before been seen.

- In 1588, Conradus Gesner published *De Piscium & Aquatilium Animantum Natura* showing hydralike monsters with multiple heads.
- In 1663, Otto von Guericke published *Protogaea*

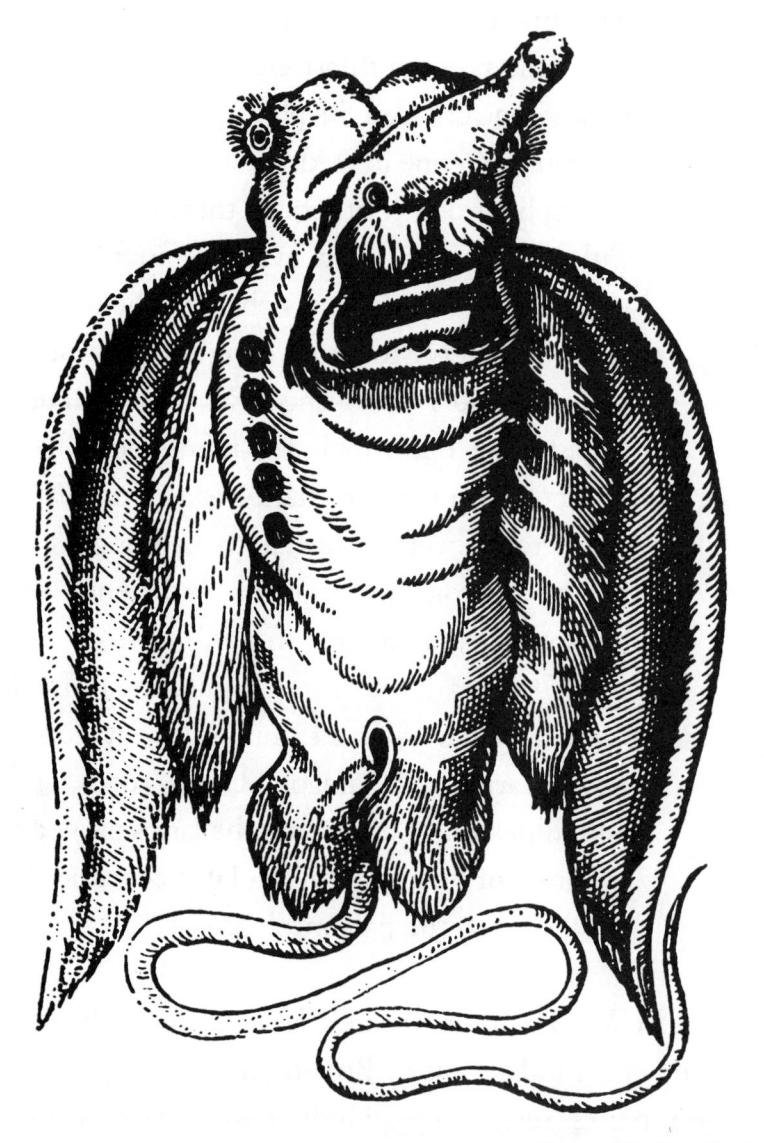

Figure 23. Sea Eagle

From Ambroise Paré, *On Monsters and Marvels*, p. 124, fig. 60.
Originally published as *Des Monstres et Prodigies*, ca. 1570.

depicting unicorn skeletons pieced together from mammoth and possibly rhinoceros remains (figure 24). (This reminds me of Odell Shepherd's remark in *The Lore of the Unicorn*: "No one in mediaeval Europe ever saw a lion or an elephant or a panther, yet these beasts were accepted without question upon evidence in no way better or worse than that which vouched for the unicorn."[4])

- In 1667, Niels Stensen, young scientist and physician to Ferdinand II, published *Canis Carchariae Dissectum Caput*. The book included monstrous illustrations of dissected giant white shark heads. For years, fossilized shark teeth were believed to be tongues of serpents turned to stone by St. Paul, and hence were named glossopetrae, or "tongue stones."

- In 1678, Anathasius Kircher published *Mundus Subterraneus* which showed numerous dragons. Chinese apothecaries used "dragon" bones, teeth, and horns to cure illnesses. (Chinese apothecaries proved invaluable to dinosaur fossil hunters in later centuries by showing fossil sites to the paleontologists.)

In William Shakespeare's *The Tempest*, published in 1623, we get an indication of British passion for paying money to see "freaks" such as a dead Indian. In the play, Trinculo studies Caliban, a feral, sullen, deformed, and complex creature, and previously the sole inhabitant of his island:

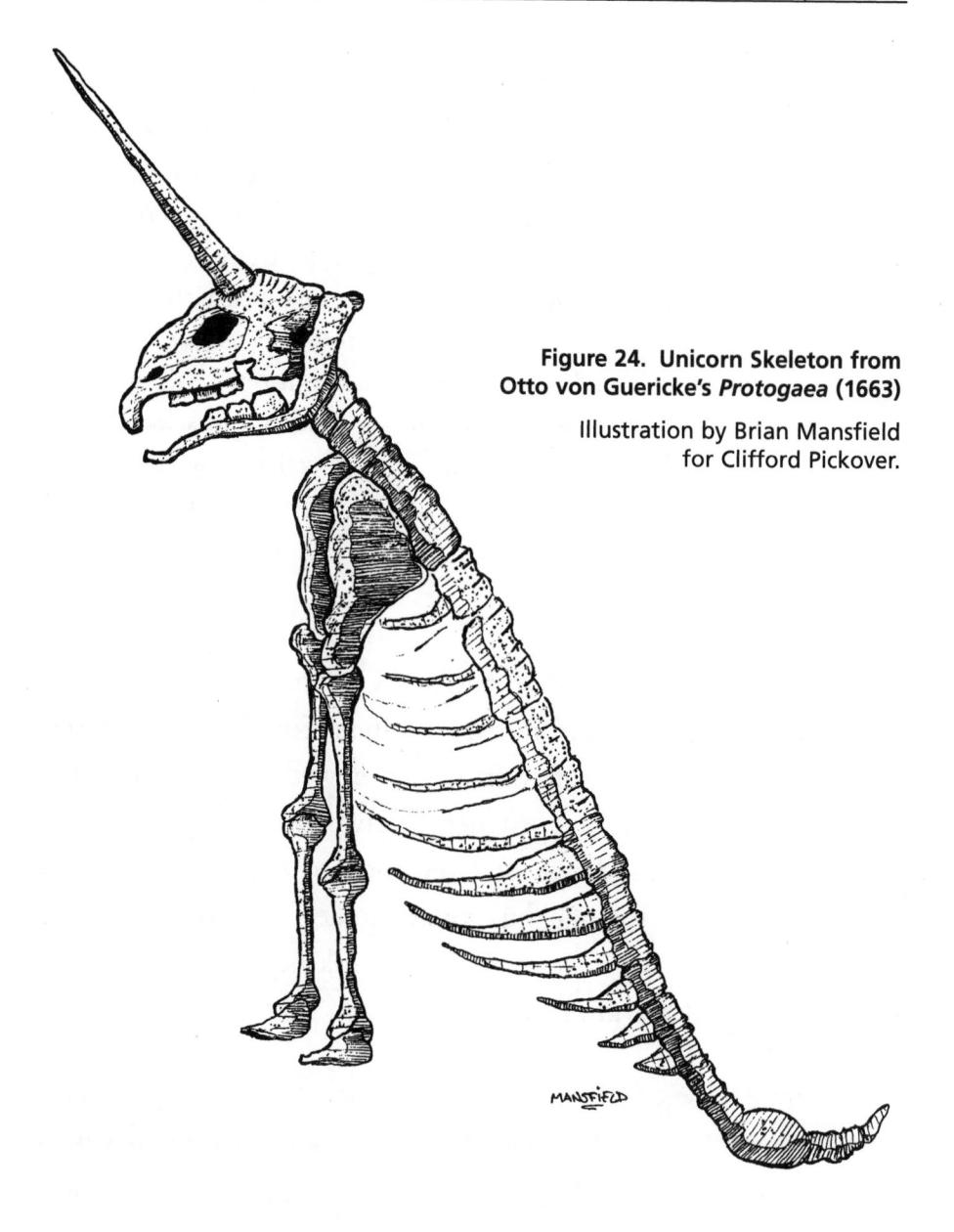

Figure 24. Unicorn Skeleton from Otto von Guericke's *Protogaea* (1663)

Illustration by Brian Mansfield for Clifford Pickover.

What have we here? a man or a fish? dead or alive?
A fish: he smells like a fish; a very ancient and fish-
like smell; a kind of not of the newest Poor-John. A
strange fish! Were I in England now, as once I was,
and had but this fish painted, not a holiday fool
there but would give a piece of silver: there would
this monster make a man; any strange beast there
makes a man: when they will not give a doit to
relieve a lame beggar, they will lazy out ten to see a
dead Indian. Legged like a man and his fins like
arms! Warm o' my troth! I do now let loose my
opinion; hold it no longer: this is no fish, but an
islander, that hath lately suffered by a thunderbolt.
(Act 2, scene 2)

The characters of Trinculo and Caliban represent the ser-
vant class alienated from their masters. For the Elizabethans,
the characters' loss of control was viewed as a threat to the
natural order and viewed negatively. Trinculo and Caliban
were without guidance and returned to their animal state.
While some of the play has comic moments, it addresses some
elements of Mary Toft's case. Is humankind, when stripped of
society's order and of rational science, nothing more than a
beast?

The fascination of Mary Toft's England for "inhuman"
creatures was also fueled by the discovery of a feral boy. While
hunting in the woods near Hamelin in Hanover, King George

I found "Peter the Wild Boy," a child of about twelve years of age. Peter's discovery took place earlier in the same year of the Mary Toft case![5] The boy knew no language and was apparently wild. All of England passionately embraced Peter's story when he was transported to England. He refused all delicacies from the royal table, preferring only raw meat and vegetables. As he developed, interest continued to grow. Jonathan Swift, author of *Gulliver's Travels*, satirized the crazed attention to the boy.

When Peter was brought to England, he was cared for by Mrs. King who housed pupils of Harrow School, including the brilliant Sir William Jones.[6] Peter also spent years on a farm in Hertfordshire where he roamed the countryside or sat before the fire—just like an amiable, dumb, neighborhood pet. Lord Monboddo, the early evolutionist, visited Peter at the farm in 1782 and found him to be a "fine specimen of unspoiled humanity."[7] Peter's guardian gave Peter a brass collar with the inscription "Peter the Wild Boy, Broadway Farm, Berkhamstead."

Peter lived to a ripe old age of about seventy-two and was eventually buried in 1785 at North Church, Hertfordshire. (See figures 25 and 26.)

Over the years, there have been many children reported to have been raised by wolves or bears, and less frequently by leopards, antelopes, goats, pigs, cattle, and sheep. Usually these children do poorly when removed from their natural set-

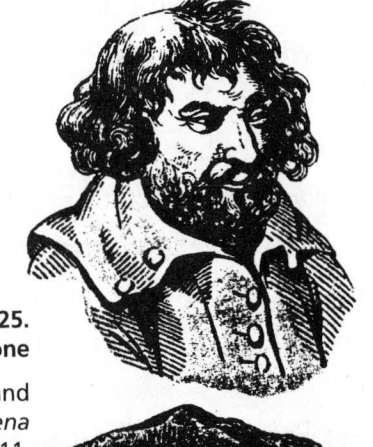

**Figure 25.
Peter the Wild Boy and His Headstone**

From John Michell and
Robert Pickard, *Phenomena*
(New York: Pantheon, 1977), p. 111.

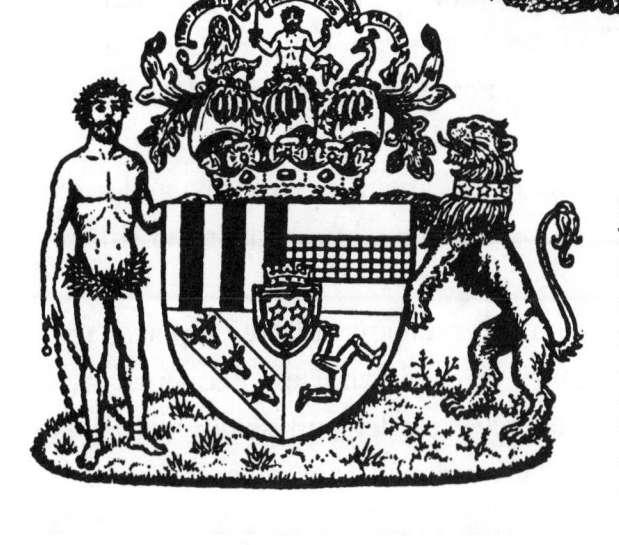

**Figure 26.
The Arms of the
Earl of Atholl**

Peter the Wild Boy,
in chains, as depicted
on the arms of the
earl of Atholl.
From John Michell
and Robert Pickard,
Phenomena, p. 111.

tings and brought into society. Instances of feral children of more than ten years of age are rarely reported, perhaps because survival in the wild is very difficult for so many years. Some of history's feral children may have actually been highly retarded children who were found wandering near animals supposed to have fostered them.[8] Autistic children have characteristics in common with those taken from "animals homes."

The simultaneous occurrence of Peter the Wild Boy and Mary Toft's babies—along with the British fascination with giants, dwarfs, bearded ladies, Siamese twins, hermaphrodites, boneless girls, mermaids, three-breasted women, and other freaks and frauds of nature—called into question what it means to be human. Creative scientists, philosophers, poets, and charlatans thrive at this shoreline. The development of Renaissance science paradoxically also illuminated the similarities between humans and nonhumans—which makes us uneasy, even today, as we consider ethical dilemmas involving animal rights and human abortion issues.

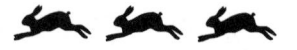

In 1726, another celebrated monster may have been on the public's mind and encouraged people to believe Mary had animal babies. In 1708, Helena and Judith, attractive and intelligent twins from Hungary, drew large crowds. They were bound together at the buttocks sharing a single vagina and rectum. Their mother believed that the deformity resulted from her viewing a two-headed dog while pregnant. Another woman with two heads and without fingers was also exhibited in London at this time.

For eighteenth-century Europeans, birth defects blurred the boundaries between human and animal, the possible and the impossible. Some Europeans saw their everyday world as only part of reality, while separated from it by diaphanous veils lay potential worlds and humans entirely different. (Go to any New Age section of a modern bookstore, and you'll see that we are still surrounded by these beliefs.)

Fascination with the freakish was not confined to England during Mary Toft's time. Dr. Honoré Fragonard (1734–1799)—a French anatomist and cousin of the French Rococo painter Jean-Honoré Fragonard—constructed sculptures from human cadavers. His cadavers were carefully skinned, preserved, and posed—and now on public view in the Fragonard Museum, which comprises three rooms of the National Veterinary School in Maisons-Alfort on the Parisian outskirts. These days, visitors to the museum (just down the river from the Charenton insane asylum, which is where some say Fragonard belonged) are struck by how much his works resemble creatures from *Alien* and other modern horror films.

Fragonard set up the museum himself in 1766, at the school where he taught. The school officials, upset by Fragonard's sickening hobby, fired him in 1771 but decided to keep the museum. His firing didn't stop Fragonard's rise to stardom among the French aristocracy who enjoyed keeping curious objects in their homes. By the time Fragonard died at the age of sixty-six, hundreds of his horrific sculptures were used to break the ice at France's finest dinner parties.[9]

Russia's Peter the Great—whose title changed from czar to emperor five years before Mary's rabbit births—had a bizarre collection of objects pickled in jars of alcohol: a man without genitals, a two-headed child, a five-footed sheep, a deformed human fetus, the organs of a hermaphrodite, and more. One of his fondest exhibits was a large pickled penis, donated to the museum by Prussia's King Frederick William. His collection also contained two human heads: one belonged to a man he suspected of being his wife's lover, and the other to a lady-in-waiting he had executed. The museum's original curator, a deformed dwarf, was eventually preserved and displayed when he died.[10]

Even the famous English surgeon John Hunter (1728–1793) had a penchant for collecting freakish things. Hunter, the founder of pathological anatomy in England, advocated experimentation in comparative biology, anatomy, physiology, and pathology. Hunter was also an enthusiastic collector of anatomical artifacts including embalmed fetuses, corpses, and skeletons. Over a period of thirty years he amassed about 66,000 specimens. His wife, Anne, complained only once, and that was when he brought home a stuffed giraffe that was too tall to fit inside the house. Hunter shortened it by chopping off the legs below the knees, and placed it in his foyer. In May 1941, the building housing Hunter's collection was bombed by the Germans, and now only 3,600 specimens remain.[11]

In addition to bizarre animal collections, there have been many hoaxes involving animals. Here are a few favorite examples:

- Just when Mary Toft was giving birth, German professor Johann Beringer published *Lithographiae Wirceburgensis*, which documented odd "fossil" finds. It all started when his teenaged assistants dug up fossil insects, spiders on their webs, lizards with intact skin, and birds with fish heads. Other fossils depicted the sun, comets, and five-pointed stars. Some contained Hebrew letters. One had "Jehovah" carved on it. Alas, Beringer was defrauded by the university's librarian and a geography professor who had carved the stones. When they learned that Beringer intended to publish his finds, they nervously warned him that the fossils were fake, but Beringer proceeded anyway. Beringer mistakenly assumed the fossils were natural and he refused to speculate further until he published his finds for colleagues to analyze.

  German Protestants in Mary Toft's day, like some modern American fundamentalists, could not believe that fossils were the vestiges of life that thrived millions of years ago. Professor Beringer suggested that many fossils were the remains of life that perished in Noah's flood, but others were "peculiar stones" carved by God as He experimented with different potential lifeforms He might create.

Beringer published his 1726 findings in Latin and illustrated them with beautiful, scholarly, engraved plates. Scientists told him he was being fooled, but he dismissed them. Just as with Mary Toft, the hoax came to an end after various confessions. Beringer's career was destroyed, and he spent his life's savings purchasing copies of his book and burning them.[12]

- In 1842 con-artist P. T. Barnum created a "Feejee Mermaid" that was displayed for "positively one week only!" at a concert hall on Broadway, New York City. Years later, Barnum recounted with amusement how he had lured the crowds to see an "ugly, dried-up, black-looking specimen about three feet long . . . that looked like it had died in great agony."[13]

- In 1845, "Dr." Albert Koch published an illustration in *Hydrarchos* depicting a "gigantic fossil reptile" 114 feet long. In actuality, Koch had pieced together the bones of five fossil whales, then showed the specimen in the United States and in England. The hoax was exposed on both sides of the Atlantic.

- The most famous "animal" hoax occurred in 1911. Charles Dawson "discovered" the Piltdown man's skull in a gravel pit near London. For decades, the skull was commonly believed to be from the earliest-known human in Western Europe. In 1953, the hoax was uncovered: someone had attached the jaw of an ape to a human skull. The jaw had been colored to make it look old, and its teeth filed to resemble human teeth. Today, the perpetrator is still unknown. Prime suspects include English anatomist Sir Arthur Keith and amateur archaeologist Charles Dawson. Some speculation has even fingered Sir Arthur Conan Doyle of Sherlock Holmes fame.[14]

Strange births involving animals and people persisted in two true-life mysteries that occurred in the early 1800s. In 1806, a terror shook the people of Leeds, England. A hen in a nearby village laid an egg that had the words "Christ is coming" inscribed on its shell. Many people visited the miracle hen and examined the wondrous eggs, convinced that the destruction of the world would soon occur. After further investigation, researchers determined that marked eggs had been cruelly forced up into the bird's body so that she would appear to lay the eggs with the messages.[15]

Even more strange is the story of Joanna Southcott (1750–1814), an English eccentric who, at age sixty-five, announced that she was expecting a child—the Second Messiah. She also said she was a virgin.

Joanna Southcott was born in Gittisham, Devon, England. She worked as a milkmaid and rejected sexual pleasure. When she was in her forties, Southcott began to hear God's voice, which allowed her to prophesy. In 1801, Joanna published the first of many books and pamphlets containing her prophecies. Her predictions attracted thousands of believers to whom she sold certificates that guaranteed them a place in heaven. She claimed God told her that only 144,000 souls would be eligible for eternal salvation. In order to guarantee her faithful a position in heaven, she issued sealed certificates bearing her oval seal in red wax.

Even after she made the startling announcement that she was pregnant with the son of "the Most High," her followers' faith did not wane. They showered her with baby gifts and an expensive crib. After October 11, 1813, she cut herself off from society to wait for the birth. Joanna wrote to every bishop and member of Parliament to tell them of the good news. On August 1, 1814, several doctors were called to check on her because she had been ill for nearly five months. The doctors concluded that she was four months pregnant.

In order to support Southcott's claims, an eminent member of the Royal College of Surgeons confirmed her pregnancy after an examination during which Joanna had remained fully clothed. She had refused to allow the physician to examine her more closely because she felt that it would be improper for the New Messiah's mother to display herself in an undignified fashion. Her apparently strong belief in her pregnancy quelled all doubts in her disciples. She believed that the world would end on October 19, 1814, the date of the rebirth of Christ.

Not everyone agreed with the physician from the Royal College of Surgeons. For example, Southcott's own physician diagnosed her as having "biliary obstructions" and attributed her excess weight to the fact that she spent all day in bed "in downy indolence." Eventually, Southcott grew frail, and on December 27, 1814, she died. On her written instructions, physicians performed an autopsy in her home—in the presence of other medical experts and a group of followers. There was no fetus within her uterus or anywhere else in her abdominal cavity.

Prior to her death, Joanna Southcott sealed a box that she said contained the secret of world peace and her predictions for the following centuries. She left instructions that the box was only to be opened in a time of national catastrophe and then only in the presence of a dozen bishops of the Church of England. In 1927, the box was X-rayed, revealing that it contained a horse pistol, dice box, purse, several books, a lottery ticket, and a night cap. Nonetheless, Southcott still has many followers today.[16]

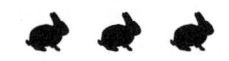

What finally became of Mary Toft? After she was released from jail, did she spend her remaining days on Earth in marital bliss? What was life like for her in prison? What happened to St. André?

Perhaps the most horrible part of Mary's story involved her treatment in prison, a facility opened to visitors. While in jail, her wardens exhibited her like a caged animal. People of all walks of life would ogle her and make dirty jokes. As I mentioned, eventually King George and his advisors grew weary of London's continuing attention and thought it best to release her from jail—although one rumor was that she had killed herself in the prison. In actuality, she spent a few months in jail and then returned to her home in Godalming.

Things quieted down after that, and I am sure Mary welcomed a more normal life. In fact, one source suggests that in February 1727 she had a normal baby.[17] The Godalming parish records identified baby Elizabeth as Mary's "first child after her pretended rabbit-breeding." This means that Mary may have actually pregnant during all of her hoaxes, a fact that may have caused physicians to believe her rabbit pregnancies were real. If this is true, it is difficult to understand how she could have endured all the probing without serious consequences to the fetus.

As the years went by, Charles, second Duke of Richmond, occasionally exhibited Mary as a curiosity at dinner parties. In 1740, Mary was tossed in jail again, this time for receiving stolen goods. In particular, she was charged with "receiving fowls at several times knowing them to be stolen."[18] In another run-in with the law she was accused of trespassing; she pleaded guilty.

A light snow gently fell when Mary Toft died on January 13, 1763, at the age of sixty. Modern historians have long searched for her gravestone. Although there are many seventeenth- and eighteenth-century Godalming stones bearing the names of the Toft family, none has ever been found for Mary herself. How and where she died and was buried is shrouded in mystery. If you ever visit southern England, please do me a favor and go to Godalming. Search the graveyards. If you find her resting place, let me know. I like to imagine a small grave stone with engraved rabbits dancing to music no one else can hear.

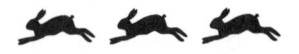

After the hoax was discovered, Nathaniel St. André's life spiraled into decline. The king and the courtiers snubbed him. He became the butt of so many jokes that many of his patients left him. His expensive tastes persisted, which soon launched him into extreme poverty. Although he retained his title of court anatomist, King George took away St. André's salary and duties.

James Douglas and Sir Richard Manningham suffered embarrassment for simply getting so involved with the affair, but their reputations and careers were largely unaffected. John Howard, midwife of Guildford, swore his innocence in the whole affair, but because he had been involved with Mary from the beginning, people were suspicious. They needed someone to blame. In early January he responded to charges that he knew about the hoax when Mary was in the bath-house, and he was fined. The charges were ultimately dropped and he retained his reputation.

Honorable Mr. Samuel Molyneux—Secretary to the Prince of Wales and St. André's companion on the Guildford trip—also bore the brunt of jokes. Luckily he was able to continue his career as courtier and politician, having married the rich daughter of the earl of Essex. In 1728, Molyneux had some kind of seizure in the House of Commons. St. André was asked to treat him, and Molyneux died a few days later. Rumors circulated that St. André had poisoned him because St. André was having an affair with Elizabeth, Molyneux's wife! This was never proven, but St. André did elope with Elizabeth Molyneux on the night of her husband's death. St. André married her, which allowed him to retire and live a comfortable life off of Elizabeth's relative wealth. Samuel Madden, Molyneux's cousin, openly accused St. André of poisoning Molyneux. Just as in today's litigious society, St. André won a court action against Madden for defamation, but rumors did not die quickly. The public viewed St. André and his wife with derision.

When Elizabeth died, her will stipulated that her wealth go not to St. André but to her relatives, leaving sad St. André in poverty once gain. He spent his remaining years in a Southampton poorhouse reminiscing about his respected, fortune-filled days as court anatomist. Nathanael St. André died in 1776 at the age of ninety-six.[19] During the last fifty years of his life, he never again ate rabbit meat.[20]

NOTES

1. Andrew Graham-Dixon, "Hogarth's Progress: What the Most Famous Artist in England Really Wanted," New Yorker (December 15, 1997): 142–51.

2. The Second Book of Esdras is an apocryphal work printed in many Roman Catholic bibles as an appendix to the New Testament. The central portion of the work, consisting of seven visions revealed to the seer Salathiel-Ezra, was written in Aramaic by an unknown Jew around 100 C.E. The book describes the future age that will succeed the present world order. The book's central theme is the justification of God's ways to man. The author, deeply concerned over the Jews' future deprived of the Temple of Jerusalem, challenges God to explain why the righteous suffer at the hands of

sinners. The answers are similar to those in the book of Job: The actions of God are inscrutable, human understanding is finite and limited, and God will always love his chosen people in spite of appearances to the contrary. The Second Book of Esdras contrasts the present, evil-ridden world to a future, heavenly age when the righteous few who survive the final judgment will live in an immortal state.

3. James Douglas's papers, as cited in Dennis Todd, *Imaginary Monsters* (Chicago: Chicago University Press, 1995), p. 43.

4. Odell Shepard, *The Lore of the Unicorn* (New York: Dover, 1993).

5. Literature reports of Peter the Wild Boy give slightly different facts. In one account, on July 22, 1724, a "naked, brownish, black-haired creature" was seen in the woods near Hamelin and later caught. In this account, it is not clear what role George I played, but it is clear that George I sent for Peter from Hanover.

6. Sir William Jones (1746–1794) was the British jurist who encouraged Westerners to become interested in Oriental studies. Of Welsh parentage, he studied at Harrow and University College, Oxford (1764–1768), and became fluent in Latin, Greek, Hebrew, Arabic, and Persian. By the end of his life, he had learned twenty-eight languages, including Chinese, often by teaching himself.

7. John Mitchell and Robert Rickard, *Phenomena: A Book of Wonders* (New York: Pantheon Books, 1977). Lord James Monboddo (1714–1799) was a Scottish jurist and pioneer anthropologist who explored the origins of language and society, and anticipated principles of Darwinian evolution. Monboddo's main work, *Of the Origin and Progress of Language*, contains curious lore on the manners and customs of primitive peoples. The book also relates

humans to the orangutan, and traces our development to a social state. Some of Monboddo's ideas and habits earned him a reputation as an eccentric; for example, he believed that children are born with tails, and at his dinner parties he strewn the table with roses in emulation of the Roman poet Horace. His sayings, whims, and oddities became legendary in his lifetime.

8. In his 1758 *Systema Naturae*, the great systematizer Linnaeus identified the wild man *Homo sapiens ferus* as a subspecies of humanity. As examples, Linnaeus cited two little boys seen by hunters among bears in the Lithuanian forests.

In 1767, hunters from Fraumark in lower Hungary followed a large bear and found human footprints leading to the bear's dens. There they found a girl of about eighteen. When taken to an asylum, she refused to eat anything but raw meat, roots, and tree bark.

Incidentally, many myths have been based on human children reared by animals. It was once respectably believed that Romulus and Remus, founders of Rome, were suckled as infants by a wolf.

9. Karl Shaw, *The Mammoth Book of Tasteless Lists* (New York: Caroll and Graff, 1998), p. 347. Neil Gaiman's recent novel *Neverwhere* has a similar theme in the 1990s. An exciting young artist embarks on a campaign of systematic grave robbery, displaying the thirty most interesting results of his depredations in glass cases. The exhibit is closed after the artist sold *Stolen Cadaver Number 25* to an advertising agency for a six-figure sum, and the relatives of *Stolen Cadaver Number 25*, seeing a photo of the sculpture in the *Sun*, sue both for a share of the proceeds and to change the title of the art piece to *Edgar Fospring, 1919–1987, Loving Husband, Father, and Uncle. Rest in Peace, Daddy.*

10. Ibid., p. 429.

11. Ibid., p. 416. Incidentally, John Hunter inoculated himself against gonorrhea and then gave himself syphilis to test his theory that they were the same disease. He was wrong. He got syphilis.

12. Martin Gardner, *Science: Good, Bad and Bogus* (Amherst, N.Y.: Prometheus Books, 1981)

13. Richard Ellis, *Monsters of the Sea* (New York: Knopf, 1994).

14. The Editors of Time-Life, *Hoaxes and Deceptions* (New York: Time-Life, 1991), pp. 124–25.

15. Charles Mackay, *Extraordinary Popular Delusions and the Madness of Crowds* (New York: Crown Publishing, 1995).

16. Ibid.

17. Jan Bondeson, *A Cabinet of Medical Curiosities* (Ithaca, N.Y.: Cornell University Press, 1997), p. 141. It is confusing to me how Mary could have had a baby in February if she actually had a miscarriage in August as reported in the literature. Perhaps Elizabeth was born prematurely? Or perhaps the August "miscarriage" wasn't a true miscarriage?

18. Quarter Sessions records at the Surrey Record Office. The Calendar of the House of Correction in Guildford in Surrey, April 15, 1740.

19. I remember the year 1776 with fondness. Not only was it the year America declared independence from England, it was also the year in which a school boy stole the jawbone of King Richard I from his tomb in at Westminster Abbey. (The tomb had a hole in it through which visitors could actually touch Richard's skull.) The jaw was kept as a family heirloom until its eventual return to the Abbey in 1906.

20. Perhaps the story of St. André never again eating rabbits is

merely a legend passed down through the generations, but would *you* eat rabbits after having delivered them, sliced up, from a woman's vagina?

CHAPTER SEVEN

SOME FINAL THOUGHTS

The rationality of our universe is best suggested by the fact that we can discover more about it from any starting point, as if it were a fabric that will unravel from any thread.
—George Zebrowski

There are two ways of spreading light: to be the candle or the mirror that reflects it.
—Edith Wharton

To be a warrior is to learn to be genuine in every moment of your life.
—Chogyam Trungpa

Human territory is defined least of all by physical frontiers.
—John Fowles, *The Magus*

COULD A MODERN MARY TOFT BE WALKING AMONG US, on the threshold of taking the entire world by storm with strange, miraculous births? Could she be your neighbor? Your boss? The teenager with a pierced tongue working at a fast-food place? The janitor in your local mall? The miniskirted temptress in the latest MTV video? A Sri Lankan priestess? A Tai Chi guru named Xena burning incense and wearing lavender in her long hair? If she gave birth to an embryonic dolphin or a hairless ape, *who* would believe her? Would *you*?

It is clear to me that medical episodes similar to Mary Toft's will recur in our modern age. The mass media—including TV, radio, newspapers and magazines—will play a pivotal role in disseminating the story, much like Fox-TV in America repeatedly aired a 1995 "documentary" purporting to be an actual autopsy of an alien found in Roswell, New Mexico. Monsters, vampires, and especially aliens are now a familiar part of our pop culture. The idea that mysterious beings are walking the planet and abducting humans with impunity has brought fame to writers such as Anne Rice, Budd Hopkins, Steven King, Dave Jacobs, Whitley Streiber, and Harvard psychiatrist John Mack who uses hypnosis to determine if people have been abducted. Recently, a teacher named Leah Haley wrote *Ceto's New Friends*, a book aimed at children ages four to eight, to teach them how to cope with their extraterrestrial visitors. On TV, *The X-Files* attracts millions of viewers. Hit movies like *Independence Day* and *Men in Black* have capitalized on the notion that our government is concealing news that it has retrieved saucer wreckage and alien bodies. Or maybe they just enjoy sci-fi as other generations did with *The Twilight Zone*, *The Outer Limits*, *One Step Beyond*, and other shows.

For those of you who have not seen the dramatic Fox-TV documentary "Alien Autopsy," imagine seeing a naked humanoid lying on an operating table in a small room. The creature has six fingers and a deep, foot-long gash in its right leg. Two humans in white contamination suits slice into its chest.

The seventeen-minute film, said to be taken in 1947, has no sound and is black and white. Although most scientists suggest the film is fake, some people still believe, or hope, that it is genuine evidence of alien life on earth. Various researchers and lay people argue about the film in magazines and on the Internet while intensely studying the footage.[1] The controversy has created a little industry. Ray Santilli, the Englishman who sold the footage, says it has been seen in over thirty-two countries. The Fox TV show debuted to surprisingly high ratings, but since then many have asked questions such as: Why does the film go so conveniently out of focus at crucial moments? Why is the camerawork so jumpy? Why hasn't the original film stock been submitted to Eastman Kodak, which has a standing offer to do a chemical analysis that would verify if it was indeed manufactured in 1947?

Most special-effects artists think the film is bogus. Many biologists have found the alien's amorphous internal organs to be implausible considering how remarkably humanoid the creature appears on the outside. The beliefs of people who think the alien is real are easily shaped by TV, books, late-night radio, and rumors on the Internet.

In 1938, many Americans became panic-stricken after listing to a realistic live radio play of *The War of the Worlds*, which depicted made-up Martians landing in Grovers Mill, New Jersey. During the play, many listeners looked out their windows and even thought they saw clear invasion signs, including flames from the battle. The incident is a testament to the remarkable power of expectation on perception.[2] The strength of expectation no doubt played a role in the Mary Toft investigations.

Here's another great contemporary hoax promoted by the media. In 1993, *The Morning Times of Laredo* published a scam of a 300-pound, 79-foot long earthworm wandering along Texas Interstate 35. Its wet body was said to leave a slimy trail and making a squishy sound as it moved. Many citizens believed the story and dared not drive Interstate 35 at night.[3]

Are you still unconvinced that today's average person

could easily be tricked into believing that a woman gave birth to rabbits? Consider this 1998 e-mail sent by a boy-scout master to an Internet mailing list (name changed to protect the innocent):

> Date: Mon, 05 Jan 1998 15:59:32-0800
> From: Rob Savant Rody
> Subject: human/animal birth?
>
> Can a human give birth to an animal (other than human)? If not, why not? The question came up in a discussion group of teens I moderate apropos artificial insemination. Frankly I had no answer, well, no explanation, rather. I'm not a biologist, just a scout master. I've taken for granted it's a biological impossibility but without any knowledge on my part to do so and it got me to thinking maybe it's not so impossible. However, I've been unable to find any literature on the subject and thought maybe someone in the Stumpers could capsule an explanation. Thanks.—Rob

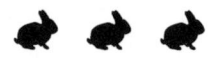

Between the fifteenth and seventeenth centuries, five hundred thousand people were burned to death and/or hanged in Europe for witchcraft and making pacts with the Devil (figure 27).[4] Other more mundane charges were often added: causing

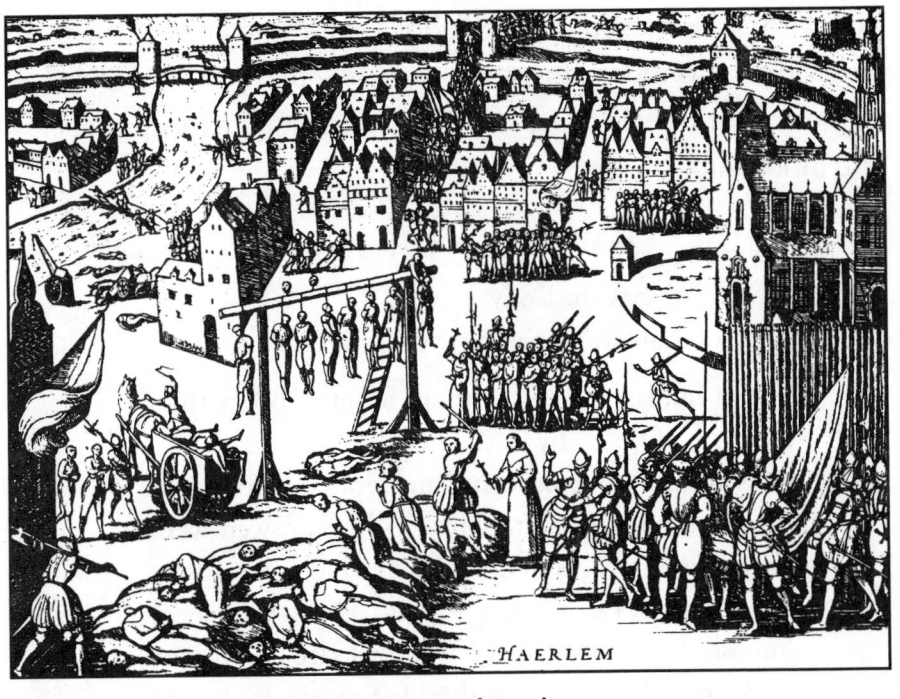

Figure 27. The Execution of the Citizens of Haarlem

This figure depicts the mass execution of the citizens of Haarlem,
who were considered disciples of the Devil. The execution,
directed by Fernando Alvarez de Toledo, Duke of Aba,
took place after the conquest of Haarlem in 1573.
From Ernst Lehner and Johanna Lehner
Picture Book of Devils, Demons, and Witchcraft, p. 78, fig. 114.

hailstorms (figure 28); ruining the crops; stealing and eating
babies. Prominent people of the day used inappropriate
methods (usually horrible torture!) to investigate charges of
witchcraft. Today we use other unsuitable methods (such as
hypnosis) to elicit "recovered" and sometimes imagined mem-

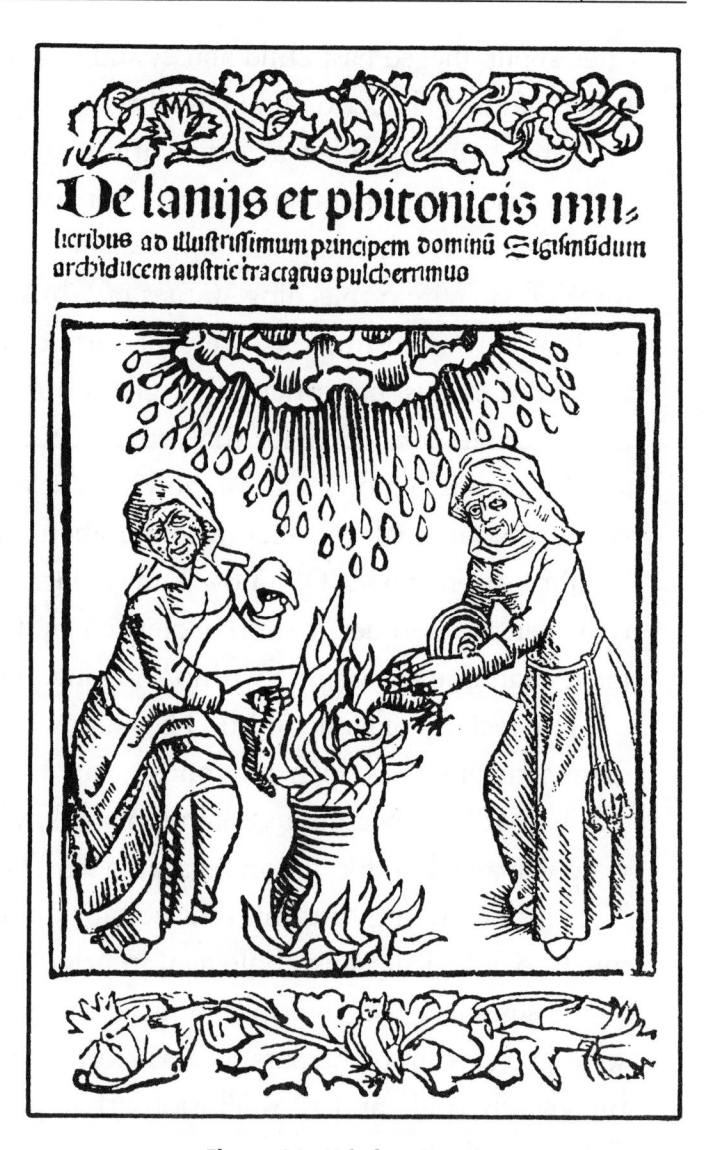

Figure 28. Witches Brewing up a Hailstorm

From Ernst Lehner and Johanna Lehner, *Picture Book of Devils, Demons, and Witchcraft*, p. 54, fig. 84. Originally published in Ulrich Molitor, *De Ianijs et Phictonicis Molieribus*, printed by Cornelius de Zierikzee, Cologne, 1489.

ories about alleged past child abuse, and to awaken "recollections" of alien abduction and past lives.[5]

After being branded as superstitions and suffering centuries of ridicule, witchcraft and other areas of the occult and supernatural (including astrology, *I Ching*, tarot, crying pictures of the Virgin, bleeding statues of Christ, demonic possession, and so forth.) have returned as respectable beliefs. Psychiatrists must be particularly vigilant not to inadvertently train patients into behavior that fits preconceptions. For example, various reports suggest how practitioners can "find" whatever they look for, such as child abuse or multiple personality disorder (MPD)—now known formally as dissociative identity disorder and characterized by the existence of more than one personality within the same individual.[6]

The recent epidemic of MPD has many causes: clinicians' diagnostic practices, such as hypnosis, that prompt patients to exhibit MPD; expectations communicated by the media; and widely available information regarding MPD's diagnostic features.[7] It is chilling to think that certain disorders may be as much sociological as psychological in origin.

In summary, we live in a bizarre and perilous age that sometimes exhibits the paranoid passion of seventeenth-century witch trials and the delusions that persisted in Mary Toft's age. Today people are accused, tried, and convicted of heinous crimes on speculative "evidence" provided by memories that did not exist until a person underwent hypnosis or was given drugs to recover "repressed" memories. The crimes excavated by the therapist include horrifying animal cruelty, incest, and satanic ritualistic abuse performed or suffered by the patient. Families are destroyed. Children are removed from homes and sometimes coaxed to confirm parents' stories. Sadly, uncritical acceptance of "recovered" memories trivializes any genuine memories of abuse and increases the suffering of real victims.[8] If Mary were alive today, could psychiatrists mistakenly use hypnosis to implant false memories of rabbit rape?

Superstitions can have other horrible consequences in our modern world. Consider the 1996 case of North Carolina state representative Henry Aldridge who explained why there was no need for his state to fund abortions for rape victims:

> People who are raped—who are truly raped—the juices don't flow, the body functions don't work, and they don't get pregnant.[9]

After Henry Aldridge's speech, the North Carolina State Legislature voted to reduce the amount of funds available to poor women having abortions from $1.2 million to $50,000. Aldridge was later appointed co-chair of the North Carolina House Committee on Human Resources, which oversees day care, services for the poor, and abortion funding.[10]

The word "hoax" is thought to be a shortening of "hocus-pocus"[11] and may range from harmless mischief to more sinister charades. *The Protocols of the Elders of Zion* is an example of the most cruel and enduring hoax. The infamous political tract justified mass murder for decades by falsely documenting an international Jewish conspiracy against the world. Fabricated by the Tsarist secret police, it helped kill 100,000 Jews in pogroms before 1919. Even though the document was exposed as a forgery in 1921, it was widely distributed by Henry Ford under the title *The International Jew*.[12] Hitler's *Mein Kampf* echoed parts of the *Protocols* as well. The evil forgery endures today, and since 1990 more than thirty editions have appeared in the U.S. alone.[13]

With many hoaxes, such as *The Protocols of the Elders of Zion*, the skeptical explanation that would expose deception is not reported by the media. Hollywood certainly likes to ignore the scientific explanations. As just one example, consider the Amityville horror—a hoax involving America's most famous haunted house located in Amityville, New York. In 1974, a man murdered his parents and siblings in the house. A year later a couple bought the house and claimed to witness many ghostly events. Subsequent investigations showed that the spooky happenings never occurred and that the murderer's lawyer concocted the horror story with the couple to make money.[14] This never stopped Hollywood from producing the horror movie *Amityville Horror: A True Story*, which many audiences believed was true.[15]

Another example of a modern hoax is spirtualism. Modern spiritualism began in 1848 when two girls, Katherine and Margaret Fox, seemed to receive ghostly messages consisting of knockings on tables. The girls traveled all over the Unites States to promote their "Spiritualist" society. Four decades later, the sisters admitted they had secretly produced the rapping sounds.

In 1917, two English schoolgirls, Elsie Wright and Frances Griffiths, created a hoax that fooled learned men for years, including Sir Arthur Conan Doyle, the creator of Sherlock Holmes. The girls took the world by storm when they showed photos of themselves with fairies dancing in Cottingley Glen, England. The 1920 Christmas issue of *Strand* magazine featured an article by Conan Doyle entitled "Fairies Photographed: An Epoch-Making Event." News of the fairies traveled far and fast, prompting Conan Doyle to tour America giving lectures about the strange phenomena. As late as 1945, fairies remained both popular and profitable for Edward Gardner, a prominent member of the theosophist movement that professed belief in wood spirits. Gardner also published a book about the girls. Sixty years after the girls took the photos, the two grown women admitted that they had simply posed with fairy cutouts in order to create the photographed scenes. People's original reaction to their photographs was a strong symbol of post-Victorian thinking: science robs the world of mystery, wonder, and beauty. British poet John Keats aptly summarizes this philosophy:

> Do not all charms fly
> At the mere touch of cold philosophy?
> There was an awful rainbow once in heaven:
> We know her woof, her texture; she is given
> In the dull catalogue of common things.
> Philosophy will clip an angels wings
> Conquer all mysteries by rule and line,
> Empty the haunted air, and gnomed mine.

The Cottingley fairy hoax gave rise to the 1997 movie *Fairy Tale: A True Story*. Arthur Conan Doyle, played by Peter O'Toole, becomes interested in the girls' story for his monthly magazine. The magician Harry Houdini, played by Harvey Keitel, sees the girls' discovery as evidence of life's spiritual dimension. In the movie's final scene, the fairies swarm around the girls' bedroom! Movie critic Sy Becker remarked, "If *Fairy Tale: A True Story* doesn't make a believer out of you, I don't know what will."

In chapter 5 we discussed more recent hoaxes, including psychic surgery, among the most dangerous of deceptions, in which practitioners pretend to remove "tumors" from peoples' bodies. These hoaxes are dangerous because patients may fail to get adequate treatment for tumors or other medical problems.

Mary Toft's story is so notable that it is actually on file at the U.S. Army Medical Library in Washington, D.C.[16] Because Mary Toft was never thought of as crazy before the incident, many accepted her tale. Even the cynical writer Alexander Pope asked a fellow scholar if he believed in the "miracle of Guildford." Some husbands did not let their wives venture out alone in the fields for fear of bunny sexual assaults.

What I have learned from Mary's legacy is that there is increasing urgency for scientists and leaders to be vigilant in their struggle against hoaxes, especially now that the mass media make it particularly difficult to distinguish fact from fiction. Hoaxes, deceptions, and truth-stretching have become a common political weapon that shapes the destinies of nations. Nonscientific reasoning and bizarre therapies are gaining acceptance as medical treatments. And the rise of racial and religious prejudices rely on the most heinous of hoaxes. The best way of battling the spread of pseudoscience is an enlightened public, able to distinguish logic from delusion, charlatans from truth-tellers.

Like St. André, today's scientists also have preconceived beliefs, expectations, and egos. That cannot be helped. However, science is not just about performing experiments, but also about *how* to perform them. It is about controlling the influence of beliefs and expectations that can color our observations and inferences. If you tell people that a guru can perform miracles, many will interpret his words with greater respect. A believer in alien abduction will interpret a light in the sky as an extraterrestrial spacecraft. A psychiatrist who believes in alien abduction will interpret a client's hypnotically facilitated ramblings differently than a psychiatrist who does not.

What will be our delusions, mysteries, and fears in the twenty-first century? Who will be the next Mary Toft?

NOTES

1. See for example, "Show Business: Autopsy or Fraud-Topsy?" *Time* 146, no. 22 (November 27, 1995). See also the Internet web page http://www. trudang.com/autopsy.html.

2. Robert E. Bartholomew, "The Martian Panic Sixty Years Later: What Have We Learned?" *Skeptical Inquirer* 22, no. 6 (November/December 1998): 40–43.

3. Ibid., p. 42.

4. Marvin Harris, *Cows, Pigs, Wars, and Witches* (New York: Vintage Books, 1974), p. 207.

5. Torture has also been frequently used in the 1900s to elicit confessions. Consider Cambodia's Pol Pot who converted a former

school to a prison. People, including children, were sent there to be tortured until they "confessed" to crimes against the state. Pol Pot had a 100 percent conviction rate and a zero percent recidivism rate. Fourteen thousand people were imprisoned there between 1976 and 1979. Only a handful survived.

6. Bertram Rothschild, "Encouraging Multiple Personality Disorder," *Skeptical Inquirer* 22, no. 6 (November/December 1998): 40–43.

7. Scott Lilienfeld, "Diagnosis and Therapy Gone Haywire," *Skeptical Inquirer* 22, no. 6 (November/December 1998): 54–55.

8. Elisabeth Loftus, "Remembering Dangerously," *Skeptical Inquirer* 19, no. 2 (March/April 1997): 20–29.

9. Christopher Cerf and Victor Navasky, *The Experts Speak* (New York: Villard, 1998), p. 14.

10. Ibid., p. 15.

11. Joe Nickell and Matt Nisbet, "CSICOP Compiles Top Ten Paranormal Hoaxes," *Skeptical Inquirer* 22, no. 4 (July/August 1998): 14–15.

12. Carl Sifakis, *The Big Book of Hoaxes* (New York: Paradox Press, 1996), p. 29.

13. Jan Willem Nienhuys, "The Top Ten Hoaxes," *Skeptical Inquirer* 22, no. 6 (November/December 1998): 66.

14. Nickell and Nisbet, "CSICOP Compiles Top Ten Paranormal Hoaxes."

15. The Amityville movie portrays a couple, played by James Brolin and Margot Kidder, who buy a house where the previous family was murdered in their sleep. When Brolin and Kidder move into the house with their two children, scary things begin to happen. Brolin slowly turns into a madman who is overly enthusi-

astic about cutting firewood with an axe. When entering the house, a priest played by Rod Steiger encounters endless problems and ailments. After a lot of horror, the family jumps into their car one night and leaves their belongings behind.

16. Sifakis, *The Big Book of Hoaxes*, pp. 72–75.

APPENDIX I

SEXUAL SUPERSTITIONS THROUGH TIME

The human body must have been designed by a civil engineer. Who else would run a sanitary line through a recreation area?

—Anonymous

And what is love without the eternal enmity between the sexes.

—Herman Hesse, *Narcissus and Goldmund*

Bisexuality immediately doubles your chances for a date on Saturday night.

—Woody Allen, *Without Feathers*

MARY TOFT'S STORY AND HER PHYSICIANS' GULLIBILITY show how "experts" can easily be coaxed into making confident pronouncements in spite of their misunderstanding and limited knowledge. Here are a few statements from learned men who freely gave their sexual wisdom and advice to the world. Notice that some of these theories deal with rabbits and the effects of maternal emotion on the developing fetus.

Imagine you are asking the questions. All of the experts' replies are based on actual quotations in the literature.[1]

"Mr. Expert, if a couple wants to make sure they have a baby *boy*, what should they do?"

- If they wish to have a male child let the man take the womb and vulva of a hare and have it dried and pulverized; blend it with wine and let him drink it. Let the woman do the same with the testicles of the hare, and let her be with her husband at the end of her menstrual period and she will conceive a male.—Tortula (physician and Professor of Medicine at the University of Salerno), *The Diseases of Woman*, ca. 1059

"Wise Sir, are birth defects caused by the mother's longing for foods?"

- Do a pregnant mother's experiences affect the off-spring? Indeed they do. The eminent Dr. Napheys reports the case of a pregnant lady who saw some grapes, longed intensely for them, and constantly thought of them. During the period of her gestation she was attacked and much alarmed by a turkey-cock. In due time she gave birth to a child having a large cluster of globular tumors growing from the tongue and exactly resembling our common grapes. And on the child's chest there grew a red excrescence exactly resembling a turkey's wattles.—Professor Oswald Squire Fowler (American, publisher, author, and lecturer on health, education, and social reform), *Sexual Science*, 1870.

"Sir, should a man over fifty years old have sexual inter-course?"

- After the "change of life" with woman, sexual congress while permissible, should be infrequent, no less for her sake than that of the husband, whose advancing years should warn him of the medical maxim: "Each time that he delivers himself to indulgence, he casts a shov-elful of earth upon his coffin."—Nicholas Francis Cooke, "Satan in Society," 1876.

"Oh Wise Ones, is masturbation normal in children?"

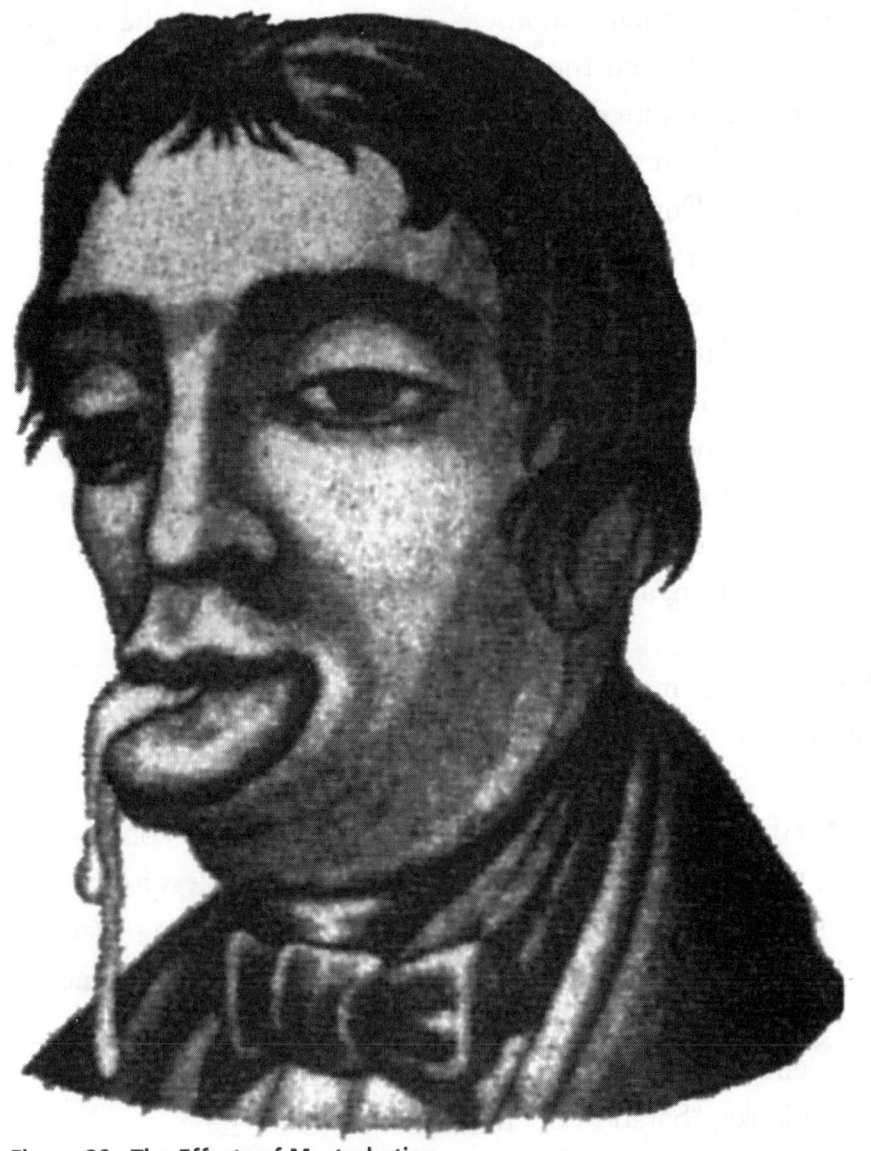

Figure 29. The Effects of Masturbation

From Christopher Cerf and Victor Navasky, *The Experts Speak* (New York: Villard, 1998), p. 17. Originally published in *The Silent Friend* (R. & L. Perry & Co., 1853).

- When the habit is discovered, it must in young children be put a stop to by such means as tying the hands, strapping the knees together with a pad between them, or some mechanical plan.—Ada Ballin (Editor of *Baby* magazine, London), *From Cradle to School: A Book for Mothers,* 1902

- When the practice of masturbation is begun at an early age, both mental and physical development may be notably interfered with. It is often stated that masturbation is a cause of insanity, epilepsy, and hysteria. I believe it to be more likely that the masturbation is the first manifestation of developing insanity.—Charles Hunter Dunn, M.D. (Instructor in Pediatrics at Harvard University and Physician-in-Chief of the Infant's Hospital), *Pediatrics: The Hygienic and Medical Treatment of Children,* 1920 (See figure 29.)

"Sir, does God think sexual intercourse is natural?"

- Let no one say that because we have these parts, that the female body is shaped this way and the male that way, the one to receive, the other to give seed, sexual intercourse is allowed by God. For if this arrangement were allowed by God, to who we seek to attain, He would not have pronounced the eunuch blessed

[Matthew 19:12].—Julius Cassianus, Gnositc Christian philosopher and leader, second century C.E.

"Sir, do women have an interest in sex?"

- If a woman is normally developed mentally, and well-bred, her sexual desire is small. If this were not so, the whole world would become a brothel and marriage and family impossible.—Joseph G. Richardson, M.D. (Professor of Hygiene at the University of Pennsylvania), *Health and Longevity*, 1909

Here are a few additional quotations to get you in the mood on those, warm romantic nights. . . .

- Sometimes in my dreams there are women. . . . When such dreams happen, immediately I remember, "I am a monk." . . . It is very important to analyze "What is the real benefit of sexual desire?" The appearance of a beautiful face or a beautiful body—as many scriptures describe—no matter how beautiful, they essentially decompose into a skeleton. When we penetrate to its human flesh and bones, there is no beauty, is there? A couple in a sexual experience is happy for that moment. Then very soon trouble begins.—Fourteenth Dalai Lama, from the *Daily Telegraph*, 1998.

- When [sexual urges] develop, I always see the negative side. There's an expression from the Nagurajuna, one of the Indian masters: "If you itch, it's nice to scratch it. But it's better to have no itch at all."—Fourteenth Dalai Lama, *Daily Telegraph.*

- It has been proven that the pig is the only homosexual animal. As this perversion is most prevalent in pork-eating nations, it is obvious that it gets into your genes through the meat.—Tasleem Ahmed, Islamic missionary from a Muslim mission in Galaway Ireland first quoted in London's *Freethinker* magazine.

- Even though they grow weary and wear themselves out with child-bearing, it does not matter; let them go on bearing children till they die, that is what they are there for.—Martin Luther, *Works* 20.84.

NOTE

1. Christopher Cerf and Victor Navasky, *The Experts Speak* (New York: Villard, 1998), pp. 11–19.

APPENDIX II

ANIMAL SUPERSTITIONS THROUGH TIME

It is only by a quirk of evolution that our sexual organs and excretory organs are united. This has led to the human race seeing sex as dirty and embarrassing. If alien sexual appendages developed in different locations, aliens would not have hang-ups, and their entire sexual psychology would be different.

  —Clifford A. Pickover, *The Science of Aliens*

The earthworm burrowing through the soil encounters another earthworm and says, "Oh, you're beautiful! Will you marry me?" and is answered: "Don't be silly! I'm your other end."

  —Robert Heinlein, *Stranger in a Strange Land*

217

Cursed be he that lieth with any manner of beast. And all the people shall say, Amen.

—Deuteronomy 27: 21

I N ADDITION TO THE EXPERTS' SEXUAL SUPERSTITIONS EXEM-plified in Appendix I, Mary Toft's predicament endured because these "experts" also had strange ideas about animals. Here are a few statements from learned men who freely gave their wisdom on the nature of animals. All of these are actual quotations in the literature[1] and include the ideas of great men such as Aristotle and da Vinci:

- Bears produce a formless foetus, giving birth to some-thing like a bit of pulp, and this the mother-bear ar-ranges into the proper legs and arms by licking it.—*The Book of Beasts* (A Latin Bestiary), twelfth century C.E.

- Bees are generated from decomposed veal.—St. Isidore of Seville (Spanish clergyman and scholar), seventh century C.E.

- Eels are not produced from sexual intercourse . . . nor are they oviparous, nor have they ever been detected with semen or ova. . . . They originated in what are called the entrails of the earth, which are found spontaneously in mud and moist earth.—Aristotle (Greek philosopher), *Parts of Animals*, 4th century B.C.E..

- When the beaver is pursued, knowing this to be on account of the virtue of its testicles for medicinal uses, not being able to flee any farther, it stops and in order to be at peace with its pursuers bites off its testicles with its sharp teeth and leaves them to its enemies.—Leonardo da Vinci (Italian scientist and artist, 1452–1519).[2]

- The lioness giveth birth to cubs which remain three days without life. Then cometh the lion, breatheth upon them, and bringeth them to life."—William of Normandy (Norman sage), thirteenth century C.E.

A few final words of wisdom:

- Animals have these advantages over man:
  they never hear the clock strike,
  they die without any idea of death,
  they have no theologians to instruct them,
  their last moments are not disturbed by unwelcome
      and unpleasant ceremonies,
  their funerals cost them nothing, and no one starts
      lawsuits over their wills.

  —Voltaire, *Candide*

- Man is the only animal that can remain on friendly terms with the victims he intends to eat until he eats them.—Samuel Butler, *Hudibras*

NOTES

1. Christopher Cerf and Victor Navasky, *The Experts Speak* (New York: Villard, 1998), pp. 334–35.

2. Ibid., p. 334.

FURTHER READING

Bartholomew, George S. Howard, and Ralph Bartholomew. *UFOs and Alien Contact: Two Centuries of Mystery*. Amherst, N.Y.: Prometheus Books, 1998.

Bondeson, Jan. *A Cabinet of Medical Curiosities*. Ithaca, N.Y.: Cornell University Press, 1997.

Broad, William, and Nicholas Wade. *Betrayers of the Truth: Fraud and Deceit in the Halls of Science*. New York: Simon and Schuster, 1982.

Cohen, Daniel. *Waiting for the Apocalypse*. Amherst, N.Y.: Prometheus Books, 1983.

The Editors of Time-Life Books. *Hoaxes and Deceptions*. Alexandria, Va.: Time-Life Books, 1991.

Frazier, Kendrick. *Science Confronts the Paranormal*. Amherst, N.Y.: Prometheus Books, 1986.

Gardner, Martin. *Fads and Fallacies in the Name of Science*. New York: Dover, 1957.

———. *The New Age: Notes of a Fringe Watcher*. Amherst, N.Y.: Prometheus Books, 1988.

———. *On the Wild Side*. Amherst, N.Y.: Prometheus Books, 1992.

———. *Science: Good, Bad, and Bogus*. Amherst, N.Y.: Prometheus Books, 1981.

———. *The Wreck of the Titanic Foretold?* Amherst, N.Y.: Prometheus Books, 1998.

Hoggart, Simon, and Mike Hutchinson. *Bizarre Beliefs*. London: Richard Cohen Books, 1995.

Klass, Philip. *UFO Abductions: A Dangerous Game*. Amherst, N.Y.: Prometheus Books, 1994.

Loewe, Michael, and Carmen Blacker. *Oracles and Divination*. Boulder: Shambala, 1981.

Mackay, Charles. *Extraordinary Popular Delusions and the Madness of Crowds*. New York: Crown Publishing, 1995. Originally published in 1852.

Marlock, Dennis, and John Dowling. *License to Steal: Traveling Con Artists, Their Games, Their Rules—Your Money*. Boulder, Colo.: Paradin Press, 1994.

Matheson, Terry. *Alien Abductions: Creating a Modern Phenomenon*. Amherst, N.Y.: Prometheus Books, 1998.

Nickell, Joe. *Wonder-Workers! How They Perform the Impossible*. Amherst, N.Y.: Prometheus Books, 1991.

Randi, James. *The Mask of Nostradamus*. Amherst, N.Y.: Prometheus Books, 1990.

———. *An Encyclopedia of Claims, Frauds, and Hoaxes of the Occult and Supernatural*. New York: St. Martin's Press, 1995.

———. *Flim-Flam*. Amherst, N.Y.: Prometheus Books, 1981.

Sifakis, Carl. *The Big Book of Hoaxes*. New York: Paradox Press, 1996.

Stein, Gordon. *The Encyclopedia of the Paranormal*. Amherst, N.Y.: Prometheus Books, 1996.

Stenger, Victor. *The Unconscious Quantum*. Amherst, N.Y.: Prometheus Books, 1995.

Thompson, Lana, and Vern L. Bullough. *The Wandering Womb: A Cultural History of Outrageous Beliefs about Women*. Amherst, N.Y.: Prometheus Books, 1999.

Todd, Dennis. *Imagining Monsters* (Chicago: Chicago University Press, 1995.

Yapp, Nick. *Greatest Hoaxes of the World*. London: Robson Books, 1992.

INDEX